Study Guide for Understanding Nursing Research
Building an Evidence-Based Practice

Eighth Edition

T0195405

Susan K. Grove, PhD, RN, ANP-BC, GNP-BC

Professor Emeritus
College of Nursing and Health Innovation
The University of Texas at Arlington
Arlington, Texas
Adult Nursing Practitioner

Jennifer R. Gray, PhD, RN, FAAN

Dean
College of Professional Studies
Oklahoma Christian University
Edmond, Oklahoma
Professor Emeritus
College of Nursing and Health Innovation
The University of Texas at Arlington
Arlington, Texas

ELSEVIER

Elsevier
3251 Riverport Lane
St. Louis, Missouri 63043

STUDY GUIDE FOR UNDERSTANDING NURSING RESEARCH, Eight edition   ISBN 978-0-323-82624-2

Notice

Practitioners and researchers must always rely on their own experience and knowledge in evaluating and using any information, methods, compounds or experiments described herein. Because of rapid advances in the medical sciences, in particular, independent verification of diagnoses and drug dosages should be made. To the fullest extent of the law, no responsibility is assumed by Elsevier, authors, editors or contributors for any injury and/or damage to persons or property as a matter of products liability, negligence or otherwise, or from any use or operation of any methods, products, instructions, or ideas contained in the material herein.

Previous editions copyrighted 2014, 2015, and 2019

Senior Content Strategist: Lee Henderson
Senior Content Development Manager: Luke Held
Senior Content Development Specialist: Maria Broeker
Publishing Services Manager: Deepthi Unni
Project Manager: Aparna Venkatachalam

Printed in the United States of America

Last digit is the print number: 9   8   7   6   5   4   3   2   1

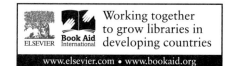

To all the nursing students, registered nurses, and advanced practice nurses who are providing evidenced based care to the many patients and families experiencing COVID.

Susan and Jennifer

To my wonderful Grandson Jack Appleton, who just turned 16 and is thinking about being a doctor.

Susan

To Birkley, Kyiah, August, Gray, and Harlan, our grandchildren. What a blessing you are to Grandy and me.

Jennifer

Preface

The knowledge generated through nursing research is rapidly expanding each year. This empirical knowledge is critical for developing an evidence-based practice in nursing that is both high quality and cost-effective for patients, families, providers, and healthcare agencies. As a nursing student and registered nurse, you will be encouraged to read, critically appraise, and use research findings to develop protocols, algorithms, and policies for practice. We recognize that research reports are complex and can be overwhelming. We developed this *Study Guide for Understanding Nursing Research* to assist you in clarifying, comprehending, analyzing, synthesizing, and applying the content presented in your textbook, *Understanding Nursing Research*, 8th edition.

The Study Guide is organized into 14 chapters, one for each chapter in the textbook. Each chapter includes learning exercises that require a range of knowledge and critical thinking skills.

In some exercises, you will define relevant terms or identify key ideas. Other exercises allow you to demonstrate comprehension of the research process by linking one idea to another. There are also exercises to increase your use of credible web-based resources to locate relevant information for classroom and clinical experiences. The most complex exercises require applying your new research knowledge by conducting critical appraisals of published quantitative and qualitative studies.

This edition of the Study Guide has been updated, refined, and condensed to include essential, current, and relevant research knowledge. The steps of the quantitative research process are explained with common research designs highlighted. The steps of the qualitative research process are also explained and compared to the quantitative research process. We have continued to include phenomenology, grounded theory research, ethnographic research, and exploratory-descriptive qualitative research.

A major emphasis is placed on critical appraisal. This Study Guide uses the revised and simplified critical appraisal processes for quantitative and qualitative research found in Chapter 12 of the textbook and included in the Guide as Appendix D. Throughout this Guide, the processes are applied to current quantitative study and qualitative study, included in Appendices A and B. Also, we have included a mixed methods study (Appendix C) that is critically appraised in selected chapters. A comprehensive appraisal of the study is provided in Chapter 14.

After you have completed the exercises for each chapter, review the answers in the Answer Key at the back of the book. Based on your correct and incorrect responses, you will be able to focus your study to improve your knowledge of each chapter's content. We believe that completing the exercises in the Study Guide will improve your performance in the classroom and during clinical experiences. We also think this Study Guide can provide you with a background for reading, analyzing, and synthesizing the evidence from research reports for application to practice.

HOW TO GET THE MOST OUT OF THIS STUDY GUIDE

The exercises in *Study Guide for Understanding Nursing Research*, 8th edition, are designed to assist you in comprehending the content in your textbook, conducting critical appraisals of nursing studies, and using research knowledge to promote an evidence-based practice.

Here are the steps that we suggest you use:

1. Read each chapter in your text before completing the chapters in this Study Guide.
2. Begin by scanning the entire chapter to get an overall view of the content.
3. Then read the textbook chapter with the intent of increasing your comprehension of each section.
4. Pay careful attention to the terms that are defined. If the meaning of a term is not clear to you, look up its definition in the Glossary and identify other pages on which the term is used in the Index at the back of the textbook.
5. Highlight key ideas in each section.

6. Examine tables, figures, and boxes as they are referenced in the text. How do they help you understand the text of the chapter?
7. Mark sections that you do not sufficiently understand. Jot down questions to ask your instructor in class or to post to your course discussion board.
8. Now, complete the Study Guide exercises; these exercises will assist you in learning relevant content.

Each Study Guide chapter includes four major headings, which are discussed as follows.

Exercise 1: Terms and Definitions

This section consists of a matching test of key terms and their definitions. Key terms are identified in color in the text and defined within the chapters to assist you in becoming familiar with essential terminology for understanding research. Being familiar with the terms will increase your ability to comprehend the course content, contribute to class or online discussions, apply your new knowledge, and critically appraise studies.

Exercise 2: Linking Ideas

This section helps you identify important information and link relevant ideas in each textbook chapter. Completing the fill-in-the-blank and matching questions will prompt you to review and analyze the content of the chapter. Reviewing and analyzing the textbook chapters are the key to comprehending and applying content related to the research process in educational and clinical activities. You may need to refer to specific sections, tables, and figures in the text to complete some of these questions.

Exercise 3: Web-Based Information and Resources

Each chapter includes questions that require searching online for answers. These questions introduce you to the wealth of information that is available online, related to research and evidence-based practice. Many of these resources are valuable websites that you may want to bookmark for use in other courses and following graduation.

Exercise 4: Conducting Critical Appraisals to Build an Evidence-Based Practice

Critical appraisal exercises are provided to give you experiences in appraising published nursing studies. In some cases, brief quotes are provided, with questions addressing information specific to the chapter content. The majority of the critical appraisal exercises focus on the three published studies that are provided in Appendices A, B, and C of this Study Guide (see Published Studies section). By completing the Study Guide, you can incorporate the critical appraisal information you have learned to perform an overall critical appraisal of these three studies. In addition, you can take the knowledge you have gained and apply it in the critical appraisal of other published quantitative, qualitative, and mixed methods studies.

Answer Key

The answers to all the questions are provided in the Answer Key in the back of the Study Guide. Restrain yourself from referring to these answers except when you are ready to check your own answers. You will learn more by reading the textbook and searching for the answers on your own.

Published Studies

Reprints of three published studies are provided in Appendices A, B, and C. The Steffen et al. (2021) study is an experimental quantitative study that is a randomized controlled trial. The Colwill et al. (2021) study is a grounded theory qualitative study; and the Greene and Ramos (2021) study is a mixed methods study focused on provider behaviors that build trust. These studies are referenced in many of the questions throughout the Study Guide. Additional published studies referenced in the Study Guide are found in the Research Article Library of the online resources for this textbook at https://evolve.elsevier.com/grove/understanding/ or can be viewed online by searching your library holdings. You are now ready to begin your adventure of learning about the research process to build an evidence-based practice.

Contents

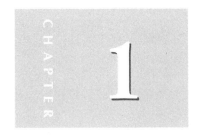

Introduction to Nursing Research and Its Importance in Building an Evidence-Based Practice

INTRODUCTION

Before completing the following exercises, read Chapter 1 in the text. The answers to these exercises are in the Answer Key at the back of the book. These exercises are designed to help you (1) learn key research terms; (2) understand the historical development of research in nursing; (3) describe how nursing knowledge is acquired; (4) identify the research methods conducted in nursing; (5) understand your role in nursing research, and (6) determine the best research evidence for practice.

EXERCISE 1: TERMS AND DEFINITIONS

Acquiring Knowledge and Research Methods

Directions: Match each term below with its correct definition. Each term is used only once and all terms are defined.

Terms

a. Borrowing
b. Case study
c. Deductive reasoning
d. Explanation
e. Inductive reasoning
f. Intuition
g. Mixed methods research
h. Nursing research

i. Outcomes research
j. Personal experience
k. Prediction
l. Qualitative research
m. Quality and Safety Education for Nurses (QSEN)
n. Quantitative research
o. Role modeling
p. Trial and error

Definitions

_____ 1. A scientific process that validates and refines existing knowledge and generates new knowledge that directly and indirectly influences nursing practice.

_____ 2. Reasoning from the specific to the general, such as reasoning from a specific symptom to the nursing diagnosis of acute pain.

_____ 3. Gaining knowledge by being actively involved in a situation, such as providing care to ventilated children in their homes.

_____ 4. A formal, objective, systematic research process to describe variables, test relationships, or examine cause-and-effect interactions among variables.

_____ 5. Reasoning from the general to the specific or from a general premise to a particular situation.

_____ 6. An approach to inquiry that combines quantitative and qualitative research methods in a single study.

_____ 7. Insight or understanding of a situation or event as a whole that usually cannot be logically explained, such as knowing that a patient's condition is deteriorating.

_____ 8. A systematic, interactive, subjective research approach used to describe cultures and life experiences from the perspective of those involved.

_____ 9. An approach with unknown outcomes that is used in a situation of uncertainty when other sources of knowledge are unavailable.

_____ 10. An in-depth analysis and systematic description of a single patient, such as a patient who survived COVID-19 after 90 days in the intensive care unit (ICU).

_____ 11. An important scientific methodology that was developed to examine the results of patient care, such as length of hospital stay, morbidity rate, mortality rate, and quality of life.

_____ 12. Knowledge generated from research that enables one to estimate the probability of a specific outcome in a given situation, such as the probability of an elderly patient falling during hospitalization.

_____ 13. Knowledge generated from research that clarifies relationships among variables.

_____ 14. Learning by imitating the behaviors of an expert, such as the process of faculty teaching students by demonstrating appropriate behaviors.

_____ 15. The appropriation and use of knowledge from other disciplines like medicine and psychology to guide nursing practice.

_____ 16. A professional nursing initiative that identified the requisite knowledge, skills, and attitudes (KSAs) for the competencies of pre-licensure education.

Evidence-Based Practice Terms

Directions: Match each term below with its correct definition. Each term is used only once and all terms are defined.

Terms
a. Best research evidence
b. Critical appraisal of research
c. Evidence-based guidelines
d. Evidence-based practice (EBP)
e. Patient circumstances

Definitions

_____ 1. The integration of best research evidence with our clinical expertise and patients' circumstances and values to produce quality health outcomes.

_____ 2. An individual's physical condition, disease trajectory, family structure, economic resources, and educational level

_____ 3. The strongest empirical knowledge available, generated from the synthesis of quality health studies to address a practice problem.

_____ 4. Rigorous, explicit clinical standards developed based on the best research evidence available in that area.

_____ 5. Careful examination of all aspects of a study to judge its strengths, limitations, credibility, meaning, and significance.

Synthesizing Research Evidence

Directions: Match each term below with its correct definition. Each term is used only once and all terms are defined.

Terms
a. Meta-analysis
b. Meta-synthesis
c. Mixed-methods research synthesis
d. Systematic review

Definitions

_____ 1. Structured, comprehensive synthesis of published quantitative studies and meta-analyses in a particular healthcare area to determine the best research evidence available for expert clinicians to use and to promote evidence-based practice.

_____ 2. Synthesis or pooling of the results from several quantitative studies using statistical analyses to determine the effect of an intervention or the strength of a relationship.

_____ 3. Systematic synthesis of the findings from independent studies conducted with a variety of methods (quantitative, qualitative, and mixed methods) to determine the current knowledge in an area.

_____ 4. Systematic compiling and integration of qualitative studies to expand understanding and develop a unique interpretation of the studies' findings in a selected area.

EXERCISE 2: LINKING IDEAS

How Research Influences Practice

Directions: The knowledge generated through research is essential to provide a scientific basis for the description, explanation, prediction, and control of nursing practice. Write a definition and provide an example of these four terms.

1. Description: _____

_____

_____

Example: _____

_____

_____

2. Explanation: _____

   _____

   _____

   Example: _____

   _____

   _____

3. Prediction: _____

   _____

   _____

   Example: _____

   _____

   _____

4. Control: _____

   _____

   _____

   Example: _____

   _____

   _____

Historical Events Influencing Nursing Research

Directions: Fill in the blanks with the appropriate word(s) or numbers.

1. _____ is considered the first nurse researcher.

2. The first research journal published in nursing was _____, which is still considered one of the strongest research journals in the profession.

3. Identify three nursing research journals that you might read to keep current in research findings.

   a. _____

   b. _____

   c. _____

4. Many national and international research conferences have been sponsored by _____ _____, the International Honor Society for Nursing, to communicate study findings.

5. The National Center for Nursing Research (NCNR) was established in the year _____ by the National Institutes of Health to promote the funding and conduct of nursing research.

6. The NCNR is now called the _____.

7. _____ is focused on the development, refinement, and use of nursing diagnoses in practice.

8. The national agency that published the first clinical practice guidelines, based on the synthesis of the best research evidence was _____ .

9. The Department of Health and Human Services (DHHS) publishes *Healthy People* documents to set health promotion goals for the US. The most recent was *Healthy People* _____ .

10. What is the name of the organization that implemented the Magnet Hospital Designation Program® for Excellence in Nursing Services? _____

Acquiring Knowledge in Nursing

Directions: Fill in the blanks with the appropriate responses.

1. List five ways of informally acquiring knowledge in nursing, and provide an example of each.

    a. _____

    b. _____

    c. _____

    d. _____

    e. _____

2. Benner's 1984 book, *From Novice to Expert: Excellence and Power in Clinical Practice*, describes the process of developing clinical expertise through which type of informal knowing? _____
_____ .

3. Identify Benner's five levels of experience in the development of clinical knowledge and expertise that are relevant today.

    a. _____

    b. _____

    c. _____

    d. _____

    e. _____

4. _____ knowledge provides an evidence base for the description, explanation, prediction, and control of nursing practice.

5. A "gut feeling" or "hunch" is an example of _____, which nurses have found useful in identifying patients' changes in health status.

6. What type of reasoning is used in the following example? _____

   Human beings experience pain.
   Infants are human beings.
   Therefore, babies experience pain.

7. Identify three important outcomes that might be examined with outcomes research.

   a. _____

   b. _____

   c. _____

8. Gordon et al. (2021) conducted a study about the experiences of nurses during the COVID-19 pandemic. "Using purposive sampling, 11 nurses from one ICU participated in semi-structured interviews. Interviews were recorded and coded; data were analyzed using content analysis" (Gordon et al., 2021, p. Abstract). Based on this excerpt, was this a qualitative or quantitative study? (The full reference is in the Answer Key.)

   _____

9. A team of researchers linked a clinical database and a financial payment database to determine the costs and length of stay for patients who had minimally-invasive back surgery. What type of research methodology did the researchers implemented? _____

10. Nurse researchers recruited participants hospitalized for sickle cell to complete three research instruments about their frequency of pain, the effectiveness of pain management, and their quality of life. The researchers statistically analyzed the data to determine the presence and strength of relationships among the variables. Was this a qualitative or quantitative study? _____

Linking Research Methods to Types of Research

Directions: Match the following research methods with the specific type of research.

Research Methods
a. Qualitative research method
b. Quantitative research method

Types of Research

_____ 1. Correlational research

_____ 2. Descriptive research

_____ 3. Ethnographic research

_____ 4. Experimental research

_____ 5. Exploratory-descriptive qualitative research

_____ 6. Grounded theory research

_____ 7. Phenomenological research

_____ 8. Quasi-experimental research

Nurses' Roles in Research

Directions: Match the levels of nurses' educational preparation with the research activities for which each group of nurses is **primarily** responsible. One activity is done by nurses with all educational preparations. <u>Use Table 1.6 from the text to guide you.</u>

Nurses' Educational Preparation

a. Bachelor of Science in Nursing (BSN)
b. Master of Science in Nursing (MSN)
c. Doctorate of Nursing Practice (DNP)
d. Doctorate of Philosophy (PhD) in Nursing
e. Post doctorate

Research Activities

_____   1. Provides clinical expertise for research teams.

_____   2. Uses research evidence in practice with guidance.

_____   3. Revises evidence-based protocols and policies for practice within a healthcare agency.

_____   4. Mentors PhD-prepared researchers.

_____   5. Critically appraises studies.

_____   6. Coordinates research teams of BSN-, MSN-, and DNP-prepared nurses.

Determining the Strength of Levels of Research Evidence

Directions: Identify the examples of research evidence by their levels of evidence, using Fig. 1.3. List the following examples of research evidence in numeric order from **I** representing the **stronget or best** evidence to **VII** representing the **weakest** evidence. You will use each level of evidence one time.

_____   Single correlational study examining the relationships of body mass index, steps walked per day, and hours spent sitting.

_____   Systematic review and meta-analysis used to develop the evidence-based guidelines for diagnosis and management of hypertension.

_____   Mixed methods research review of qualitative and quantitative studies about effectiveness of medication administration technologies on medication errors.

_____   Random controlled trial of a new medication for persons with Type 2 diabetes.

_____   Opinions of respected authorities on the management of patients with COVID-19 and sickle cell disease.

_____   Single qualitative study of the process of weaning older adult patients from mechanical ventilation.

_____   Quasi-experimental study of a nursing intervention for managing anxiety in anxious young adults.

EXERCISE 3: WEB-BASED INFORMATION AND RESOURCES

Directions: Answer the following questions with the appropriate website or relevant information.

1. On the website of the National Institute of Nursing Research (NINR), find the Milestones in NINR History page. In 1994, what was the name of the researcher who tested culturally-sensitive interventions to reduce sexual risk behaviors related to HIV among vulnerable populations?

_____

_____

_____

2. In May 2021, the Agency for Healthcare Research and Quality (AHRQ) released a Special Emphasis Notice requesting health services research grant applications for evidence-based interventions related to what topic? The topic is one of the nation's goals related to healthcare services.

_____.

3. The National Coalition for Hospice and Palliative Care revised their clinical practice guidelines in 2018. What edition was this of the guidelines? _____

   What is the website where you can download a copy?

_____

4. Identify the URL for Evidence-Based Resources for Social Determinants of Health on the current *Healthy People* website. _____

5. Identify one of the social determinants of health listed on the page identified in Question 4. _____

_____

6. Search for Quality and Safety Education for Nurses (QSEN) Competencies and locate those for pre-licensure nursing education. What is the definition of the Evidence-Based Practice (EBP) Competency?

_____

_____

7. Compare the QSEN EBP competency and the text's definition of EBP.

_____

EXERCISE 4: CONDUCTING CRITICAL APPRAISALS TO BUILD AN EVIDENCE-BASED PRACTICE

Directions: Locate the research articles in Appendices A, B, and C of the Study Guide. In the subsequent chapters of the text, you will find guidelines for critically appraising different aspects of studies.

The title, abstract, and researchers (authors) are the focus of these questions. Think of yourself as a detective looking for clues about the study in the title and abstract. Look at the credentials and affiliations (employers) of the researchers to evaluate their background and qualifications.

Steffen et al. (2021) Study

1. According to the title, participants in the study had which two medical conditions? _____ _____

2. When were the data collected? _____

3. How many of the researchers had earned a doctoral degree? _____

4. How many participants were in the motivational interviewing group? _____

5. If you wanted to contact the researchers, to whom do you address the correspondence? _____

Colwill et al. (2021) Study

This article does not have an abstract.

1. How many of the authors were nurses? _____

2. Based on the mailing address of the corresponding author and other clues related to the authors, in which hospital do you think this study was conducted? _____

3. Which type of qualitative research was implemented for the study? _____

4. As the result of intravenous drug use/abuse, what medical condition did the participants have? _____ _____

5. The article was published in which journal? _____

Greene and Ramos (2021)

1. The quantitative portion of the study included a secondary analysis of data from a _____ survey.

2. How many interviews were conducted? _____

3. According to the abstract, the survey sample had how many participants? _____

4. Greene is affiliated with a university in which US state? _____

5. In the quantitative study, trust in one's healthcare provider was high correlated with how many survey items? _____

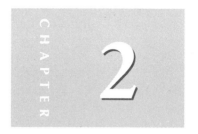

Introduction to Quantitative Research

INTRODUCTION

You need to read Chapter 2 and then complete the following exercises. These exercises will assist you in (1) learning the steps of the quantitative research process; (2) identifying the different types of quantitative research (descriptive, correlational, quasi-experimental, and experimental) in the nursing literature; and (3) reading quantitative research reports. The answers for the following exercises are in the Answer Key at the back of the book.

EXERCISE 1: TERMS AND DEFINITIONS

Directions: Match each term below with its correct definition. Each term is used only once and all terms are defined.

Terms

a.	Applied or clinical research	k.	Pilot study
b.	Assumptions	l.	Quantitative research
c.	Basic research	m.	Quasi-experimental research
d.	Control	n.	Reading a research report
e.	Correlational research	o.	Research framework
f.	Descriptive research	p.	Research problem
g.	Design	q.	Research purpose
h.	Generalization	r.	Sampling
i.	Interpretation of research outcomes	s.	Setting
j.	Limitations	t.	Variables

Definitions

_____ 1. Formal, objective, rigorous, systematic process for generating information about the world from numerical data that describes, tests relationships, and examines cause-and-effect interactions among variables.

_____ 2. Location for conducting research that can be natural, partially controlled, or highly controlled.

_____ 3. Scientific investigations conducted to generate knowledge that will directly influence or improve nursing practice.

_____ 4. Imposing of rules by the researcher to decrease the possibility of error and increase the probability that the study's findings are an accurate reflection of reality.

_____ 5. Process of selecting participants that are representative of the population being studied.

_____ 6. Use of a variety of critical thinking skills, such as skimming, comprehending, and analyzing to facilitate an understanding of a study.

_____ 7. Extension of the implications of the findings from the sample that was studied to the larger population.

_____ 8. Smaller version of a proposed study conducted to develop and/or refine the methodology, such as the intervention, measurement methods, or data collection process, to be used in a larger study.

_____ 9. The specific goal or focus of a study that directs the remaining steps of the research process.

_____ 10. Restrictions in a study methodology and/or research framework that may decrease the credibility and generalizability of the findings.

_____ 11. Type of quantitative research that is conducted to examine causal relationships or to determine the effect of an independent variable on the dependent variable, but lacks the control of an experimental study.

_____ 12. Investigations conducted to increase knowledge or understanding of the fundamental aspects of phenomena and of observable facts without specific applications towards processes or products; the pursuit of knowledge for knowledge's sake that is sometimes referred to as bench research.

_____ 13. Type of quantitative research that involves the exploration of phenomena in real-life situations.

_____ 14. Concepts at various levels of abstraction that are measured, manipulated, or controlled in a study.

_____ 15. Statements that are taken for granted or are considered true even though they have not been scientifically tested.

_____ 16. Plan or blueprint for conducting a study that maximizes control over factors that could interfere with the study's desired outcome.

_____ 17. Type of quantitative research that involves the systematic investigation of associations between or among variables.

_____ 18. A step in the research process that identifies the gap in nursing knowledge needed for practice and indicates an area for further research.

_____ 19. Step in the research process that involves exploring the significance of the findings, forming conclusions, considering implications for nursing, and suggesting further studies.

_____ 20. The abstract, theoretical basis for a study that enables the researcher to link the findings to nursing's body of knowledge.

EXERCISE 2: LINKING IDEAS

Control in Quantitative Research

Directions: Fill in the blanks with the appropriate word(s).

1. Basic research is usually conducted in a(n) _____setting.

2. _____ and _____ studies are usually conducted in natural settings and are not controlled to the same degree as other types of quantitative research.

3. Extraneous variables need to be controlled in _____ and _____ _____ types of quantitative research to ensure that the findings are accurate and not the result of bias or errors.

4. Randomized controlled trials (RCTs) should include _____ assignment of study participants to the intervention and control groups.

5. Frequently, a(n) _____ sampling method is used in descriptive and correlational studies. However, a(n) _____ sampling method might also be used.

6. A study participant's home is an example of a(n) _____ setting.

7. Applied research is usually conducted in _____ or _____ _____ settings.

8. Researcher control is greatest in what type of quantitative study? _____

9. Hospital units are examples of _____ settings that allow the researchers to control some of the extraneous variables in the study.

10. Quantitative studies that include interventions are _____ and _____.

Steps of the Research Process

Directions: Fill in the blanks with the appropriate word(s).

1. The research process is similar to the _____ and the _____ process.

2. List the steps of the quantitative research process in their typical order of occurrence.

Step 1 _____

Step 2 _____

Step 3 _____

Step 4 _____

Step 5 _____

Step 6 _____

Step 7 _____

Step 8 _____

Step 9 _____

Step 10 _____

Step 11 _____

_____

_____

3. Identify three common assumptions on which various nursing studies have been based.

   a. _____

   b. _____

   c. _____

4. Identify four reasons for conducting a pilot study.

   a. _____

   b. _____

   c. _____

   d. _____

5. Koyuncu et al. (2021, p. 200) examined the effect of family presence on stress response after bypass surgery and reported: "Environmental stress factors such as noise, lights, bad odors, and the presence of other patients in the ICU [intensive care unit] environment could not be standardized." In a research report, these are examples of _____. (The complete citation for this study is in the Answers section.)

Reading Research Reports

Directions: Fill in the blanks with the appropriate responses.

1. The most common sources for nursing research reports are professional journals. Identify three nursing research journals.

   a. _____

   b. _____

   c. _____

2. Identify two clinical journals that include several research articles in each issue.

   a. _____

   b. _____

3. Identify four major or primary sections of a research report.

   a. _____

   b. _____

   c. _____

   d. _____

4. Identify four elements or steps of a quantitative research process that are included in the Methods section of a research report.

   a. _____

   b. _____

   c. _____

   d. _____

5. The Discussion section ties the other sections of the research report together and gives them meaning. Identify five elements or components that are included in this section of a research report.

   a. _____

   b. _____

   c. _____

   d. _____

   e. _____

6. The problem and purpose are often identified in the _____ section of a research report.

7. The reference list at the end of a research report includes the relevant _____ and _____ sources that provide a basis for the study and are cited in the report.

8. Reading a research report involves _____, _____, and _____ the content of the report.

9. In reading a research report, the comprehending step involves _____ _____.

10. In reading a research report, the analyzing step involves _____ _____.

Types of Quantitative Research

Directions: Match the type of quantitative research listed below with the examples of study titles. The types of quantitative research are used more than once.

Type of Quantitative Research

   a. Descriptive research
   b. Correlational research
   c. Quasi-experimental research
   d. Experimental research

Examples of Study Titles

_____ 1. Exploring the incidence, hospitalization, and mortality rates for COVID-19 patients in the United States (US) for 2020.

_____ 2. Determining the associations of risky behaviors of adolescents and young adults with sexually transmitted diseases.

_____ 3. Examining the links among age, gender, knowledge of AIDS, and use of condoms by college students.

_____ 4. Examining the effect of impaired physical mobility on skeletal muscle atrophy in laboratory rats.

_____ 5. Comparing the COVID-19 immunization rates for different US states.

_____ 6. Determining the effects of a relaxation technique versus standard care on patients' postoperative pain and anxiety levels in a day surgery center.

_____ 7. Determining the quality of life of family caregivers of older adults with Alzheimer's disease.

_____ 8. Examining the relationships among hardiness, depression, and coping in institutionalized older adults.

_____ 9. "Effect of family presence on stress response after bypass surgery" (Koyuncu et al., 2021, p. 193).

_____ 10. Examining the relationships among the lipid values, blood pressure, weight, and hours of computer use for adolescents.

_____ 11. Determining the effect of warm and cold applications on the resolution of intravenous (IV) infiltrations in hospitalized patients.

_____ 12. Comparing the ages of mothers pregnant with their first child in three racial groups (African American, Caucasian, and Hispanic).

_____ 13. Examining the association of age, weight, chronic diseases, and length of stay in the ICU for patients with COVID-19.

_____ 14. Exploring the use of robotic technology in pediatric care.

_____ 15. Determining the effectiveness of an automated educational intervention on ICU nurses prevention of delirium in critically ill adults.

EXERCISE 3: WEB-BASED INFORMATION AND RESOURCES

Directions: Search for quantitative study information.

1. During recent years, extensive basic or bench research has been conducted in the United States to describe human genetics.

    a. Identify the national institute involved in this research: _____

    _____

    b. Identify the website for this national institute: _____

_____

    c. Identify the website for funding provided by this institute: _____

_____

    d. Genomic research began with what project? _____

_____

2.

    a. Identify the website for the National Institute of Nursing Research (NINR): _____
        Search this web page and examine the types of research being conducted in nursing.

    b. Identify the website for the NINR "Research Funding Opportunities": _____

_____

    c. Identify the website for the NINR Mission and Strategic Plan for 2021 to 2026 that is under development:

_____

3. Identify the website that presents the findings and reports of the studies funded by the Agency for Healthcare Research and Quality (AHRQ): _____

_____

4. Determine the website for the Centers for Disease Control and Prevention (CDC): _____

5. What is the main disease identified on the CDC website? _____

EXERCISE 4: CONDUCTING CRITICAL APPRAISALS TO BUILD AN EVIDENCE-BASED PRACTICE

Directions: Read the research articles in Appendices A, B, and C and answer the following questions.

Type of Quantitative and/or Qualitative Research

Directions: Identify the type of quantitative and/or qualitative research conducted in each study. You will not use all the answers.

Type of Quantitative and Qualitative Research

a. Descriptive research
b. Correlational research
c. Quasi-experimental research
d. Experimental research

e. Phenomenological research
f. Grounded theory research
g. Exploratory-descriptive research
h. Ethnographic research

Study

_____ 1. Steffen, P. L. S., Mendonça, C. S., Meyer, E., & Faustino-Silva, D. D. (2021). Motivational interviewing in the management of Type 2 diabetes mellitus and arterial hypertension in primary health care: An RCT. *American Journal of Preventive Medicine, 60*(5), e203–e212. (Provided in Appendix A)

_____ 2. Colwill, J. P., Sherman, M. I., Siedlecki, S. L., & Siegmund, L. A. (2021). A grounded theory approach to the care experience of patients with intravenous drug use/abuse-related endocarditis. *Applied Nursing Research, 57*, Article 151390. (Provided in Appendix B)

_____ 3. Greene, J., & Ramos, C. (2021). A mixed methods examination of health care provider behaviors that build patients' trust. *Patient Education and Counseling, 104*, 1222–1228. (Provided in Appendix C)

Type of Setting

Directions: Identify the type of setting for each study and provide rationales for your answers.

a. Natural setting
b. Partially controlled setting
c. Highly controlled setting

_____ 1. Steffen et al. (2021) study setting: _____

Rationale: _____

_____

_____

_____ 2. Colwill et al. (2021) study setting: _____

Rationale: _____

_____

_____

_____ 3. Greene and Ramos (2021) study setting: _____

Rationale: _____

_____

_____

Type of Research Conducted (Applied or Basic)

Directions: Indicate the type of nursing research conducted in each study.

Type of Nursing Research

a. Applied nursing research
b. Basic nursing research

Study

_____   1. Steffen et al. (2021) study

_____   2. Greene and Ramos (2021) study

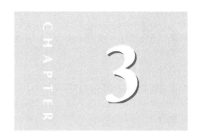

CHAPTER 3

Introduction to Qualitative Research

INTRODUCTION

Read Chapter 3 and then complete the following exercises. These exercises will assist you in learning key terms and reading, comprehending, and critically appraising published qualitative studies. The answers for the following exercises are in the Answer Key at the back of the book.

EXERCISE 1: TERMS AND DEFINITIONS

Directions: Match each term below with its correct definition. Each term is used only once and all terms are defined.

Definitions Related to Qualitative Research

Terms

a. Audit trail
b. Bracketing
c. Dwelling with the data
d. Ethnographic research
e. Ethnonursing research
f. Exploratory-descriptive qualitative research
g. Field notes
h. Focus group
i. Grounded theory research
j. Member checking

k. Methodology
l. Moderator or facilitator
m. Phenomena
n. Phenomenological research
o. Probes
p. Rigor
q. Saturation
r. Social constructivism
s. Transcription
t. Unstructured interview

Definitions

_____ 1. Research based on a pragmatic philosophy and focused on increasing understanding or finding a solution.

_____ 2. Typing a verbatim narrative from a recorded interview or focus group.

_____ 3. A person selected to guide the discussion of a focus group and may share characteristics of focus-group members.

_____ 4. Qualitative method that describes social processes and proposes a framework of related concepts.

_____ 5. The strength and credibility of a qualitative study produced by implementing appropriate study methods.

_____ 6. Follow-up statements or questions made by the researcher to obtain more information from the participant.

_____ 7. Gathering data from multiple participants simultaneously to encourage interaction and discussion.

_____ 8. Research term that refers to a general type of research, such as qualitative research.

_____ 9. Using Dr. Leininger's methods to describe a cultural group.

_____ 10. Notes from a research observation.

_____ 11. Setting aside one's values and perspectives during the data collection and analysis process.

_____ 12. Providing a participant a copy of the transcript, summary, or initial analysis of an interview to ensure the researcher understood.

_____ 13. Philosophy that a person's beliefs and actions are based on the shared reality developed through actions with others.

_____ 14. The point in data collection and analysis when additional participants do not provide new information.

_____ 15. Questioning research participants orally without a fixed set of questions.

_____ 16. Study of cultures based on anthropology.

_____ 17. Conscious awareness of experiences that comprise being alive.

_____ 18. Researcher spends considerable periods of time reading and reflecting on the data.

_____ 19. A record of decisions made during data collection, analysis, and interpretation.

_____ 20. Studies focused on the lived experience.

Definitions Related to Ethnography

Terms
a. Critical ethnography
b. Emic approach
c. Etic approach
d. Focused ethnography
e. Going native
f. Immersion
g. Key informant

Definitions

_____ 1. Type of study that explores the culture of a specific group of people or an organization for a shorter time.

_____ 2. Gaining familiarity with the aspects of a culture by spending time in it.

_____ 3. A person with extensive knowledge and influence in a culture who may facilitate the work of an ethnographer.

_____ 4. Studying a culture using an insider perspective that recognizes the uniqueness of the individual.

_____ 5. Studying a culture using the perspective of a naive outsider.

_____ 6. A researcher becomes a part of the culture and loses the ability to objectively observe.

_____ 7. Type of study that examines the political and socio-ecological factors of a culture.

Definitions in Your Own Words

Directions: Define the following terms in your own words without looking at your textbook. Then check your definitions with those in the glossary of your textbook. Using this strategy, you can identify elements of the term that are not yet clear in your mind. Reread that section of the chapter to clarify your understanding of the term.

1. Observation: _____

_____

_____

2. Coding: _____

_____

_____

3. Researcher-participant relationship: _____

_____

_____

EXERCISE 2: LINKING IDEAS

People and Their Contributions to Qualitative Research

Directions: Match the names of people below with the correct description. Each name is used only once and all people are described.

Description
a. Philosopher associated with the interpretive approach to phenomenology
b. Developed the Sunshine Model of Transcultural Nursing Care
c. Philosopher associated with the descriptive approach to phenomenology
d. Their early studies on dying led to the grounded theory method

Names

_____ 1. Glaser and Strauss

_____ 2. Heidegger

_____ 3. Husserl

_____ 4. Leininger

Qualitative Research Methodology

Directions: Fill in the blanks with the appropriate word(s).

1. During a phenomenological study, the researcher listens to the recordings of interviews several times and reads and rereads the transcripts to _____ with the data.

2. An ethnographer lives in a different culture for a year, learns the language, and slowly stops communicating with family and friends in her home country. When asked when she plans to return, the ethnographer says she has not decided because she prefers the culture here more than she does the culture of her own country. There is a danger that the ethnographer has "gone _____."

3. The observer writes down side comments, conditions in the environment, and descriptions of body language during the focus group. The observer is preparing _____.

4. During a grounded theory study of families after the loss of a family member to COVID-19, the researcher continues to recruit participants until _____ is reached, defined as additional participants not providing new information.

5. The researcher begins unstructured interviews with a general question to allow participants to tell their experiences of being diagnosed with lung cancer. If a participant stops talking and seems unable to continue, the researcher has prepared short questions to help the participant continue or add new information. These questions are called _____.

Approaches to Qualitative Research

Directions: Match each qualitative approach with its characteristics. Label them P, G, E, and/or EDQ according to the key below for each area. All answers will be used at least once and some more than once.

Qualitative Approach

P = Phenomenological research   E = Ethnographic research
G = Grounded theory research   EDQ = Exploratory-descriptive qualitative research

Characteristics

_____ 1. Seeks to develop a framework of concepts or theory.

_____ 2. May use key informants in the study of cultures.

_____ 3. Refers to a philosophy and a research method.

_____ 4. Emerged from the discipline of anthropology.

_____ 5. Often based on a pragmatic philosophy.

_____ 6. Interested in the social processes.

_____ 7. Studies the meaning of a lived experience.

_____ 8. Undertaken to solve a problem or obtain information to use to improve a service.

EXERCISE 3: WEB-BASED INFORMATION AND RESOURCES

1. Identify the names, publishers, and URLs of at least 3 journals that publish primarily qualitative research. The URL needs to provide a description of what the journal publishes. You may find the names through your university's library databases and search for the URL through an internet search engine, such as Google. Complete the table with the information that you find.

Journal Name	Publisher	URL

2. What can you learn about a qualitative study from reading the title and the abstract and skimming the article?

_____

_____

Follow this link to an open access journal with a qualitative nursing research study that you will use to complete this question.

Nasrabadi, A., Wibisono, A., Allen, K., Yaghoobzadeh, A., & Bit-Lian, Y. (2021). Exploring the experiences of nurses' moral distress in long-term care of older adults: A phenomenological study. https://bmcnurs. biomedcentral.com/articles/10.1186/s12912-021-00675-3

Directions: Read the title and the abstract and skim the article. Then complete the information in the table.

Study Characteristic	Answer
Country in which the study was conducted.	
Identify the qualitative approach conducted (phenomenology, grounded theory, exploratory-descriptive qualitative, ethnography research).	

Identify the human experience or topic of the study.	
Describe the sample, including the total number, number of males, number of females, average age, and average number of years of job experience.	
How were the data collected?	

3. Surprisingly, the U.S. National Park Service has a website for distance education that includes a section on ethnographic research. Go to this website (https://www.nps.gov/ethnography/aah/aaheritage/ERCa.htm) to answer two questions.
   a. Provide one of the definitions of ethnographic research in the first paragraph of the section, "What is Ethnographic Research?"

   _____

   _____

   _____

   _____

   b. According to the website, who conducts ethnographic research?

   _____

   _____

   _____

4. Identify 2 websites on which you found podcasts about qualitative research.

   _____

   _____

EXERCISE 4: CONDUCTING CRITICAL APPRAISALS TO BUILD AN EVIDENCE-BASED PRACTICE

Directions: Read the Colwill et al. (2021) article in Appendix B of this study guide. Answer the following questions about the study that are from the Critical Appraisal Guidelines in Chapter 3.

1. What qualitative methodology was implemented in this study? _____

   _____

2. Was the outcome of the study as presented in the research report appropriate for the methodology?

   _____

   _____

3. Were the following sections clear, concise, and complete in the research report: Introduction, Methods, Results, and Discussion?

   _____

   _____

   _____

   _____

   _____

   _____

   _____

4. Were the steps of the study clearly identified? Briefly describe each step of the study, using Table 3.1 in the Grove and Gray (2023) research textbook.

   _____

   _____

   _____

   _____

   _____

   _____

   _____

5. Were any of the steps of the research process missing? If so, which one(s)?

    _____

    _____

6. The data were collected through interviews. Did the interview questions address concerns expressed in the research problem? Explain your answer.

    _____

    _____

    _____

7. Were the interview questions relevant for the study purpose and objectives or questions? Explain your answer.

    _____

    _____

    _____

8. Were the interviews adequate in length and number to address the research purpose and answer the research question?

    _____

    _____

9. Were data analysis and interpretation consistent with the philosophical orientation, research problem, research question, purpose, and methodology of the study? Explain your answer.

    _____

    _____

    _____

    _____

10. Did the researchers describe how they recorded decisions made during analysis and interpretation? Explain your answer.

    _____

    _____

    _____

11. Did the researchers link the codes and themes used with participants' quotations? Provide one example.

_____

_____

_____

_____

12. Did the researchers provide adequate description of the data analysis and interpretation processes? Explain your answer.

_____

_____

_____

_____

Directions: Read the Greene and Ramos (2021) article in Appendix C of this study guide. Answer the following questions about the qualitative component of this mixed methods study.

13. How were the qualitative data collected for this study? How many qualitative participants were there in the study?

_____

_____

14. Was the data collection and analysis adequate to meet the purpose of the qualitative part of the study?

_____

_____

_____

_____

15. What were the key dimensions of trust of the participants' usual healthcare providers? Provide an example of a quotation that supported one of the dimensions.

_____

_____

_____

_____

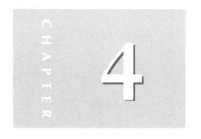

Examining Ethics in Nursing Research

CHAPTER 4

INTRODUCTION

You need to read Chapter 4 and then complete the following exercises. These exercises will assist you in understanding and critically appraising the ethical aspects of a variety of nursing studies. The answers for these exercises are in the Answer Key at the back of the book.

EXERCISE 1: TERMS AND DEFINITIONS

Directions: Match each term below with its correct definition. Each term is used only once and all terms are defined.

Terms

a. Anonymity	k. Ethical principles
b. Autonomy	l. Identifiable private information
c. Benefit–risk ratio	m. Informed consent
d. Broad consent	n. Institutional review board (IRB)
e. Coercion	o. Nontherapeutic research
f. Comprehension	p. Plagiarism
g. Confidentiality	q. Privacy
h. Deception	r. Research misconduct
i. Disclosure	s. Therapeutic research
j. Discomfort and harm	t. Voluntary agreement

Definitions

_____ 1. Research conducted to generate knowledge for a discipline; the results might benefit future patients, but will probably not benefit the research subjects.

_____ 2. Potential participant receives information about a study, agrees to participate, and signs a document to that effect.

_____ 3. Potential study participants understand the information provided to them.

_____ 4. Condition in which a subject's identity cannot be linked, even by the researcher, with his or her individual responses.

_____ 5. Freedom of an individual to determine the time, extent, and general circumstances under which private information is shared.

_____ 6. Anticipated or actual physical, emotional, social, or economic risks associated with a study.

_____ 7. Potential participant gives researchers permission to store, maintain, and use indentifiable specimens or private information for other studies.

_____ 8. A committee of peers that approves, disapproves, or requests changes to a study after examining a study for ethical concerns.

_____ 9. The balance between potential benefits and risks in a study that must be weighed by researchers to promote the conduct of ethical research.

_____ 10. One person threatens another with harm or offers an excessive reward to obtain compliance.

_____ 11. Practices such as fabrication, falsification, or forging of data; dishonest manipulation of the study design or methods; and plagiarism.

_____ 12. Potential participants agree to be in a study of their own volition.

_____ 13. Actually misinforming participants for research purposes.

_____ 14. Research that provides a patient with an opportunity to receive an experimental treatment that might have beneficial results.

_____ 15. Principles of respect for persons, beneficence, and justice, which are relevant to the conduct of research.

_____ 16. Researcher manages participants' data in way that keeps the data private from others.

_____ 17. Providing understandable and relevant information about a study to a potential participant

_____ 18. Any information, including demographic information, collected from an individual that is created or received by healthcare providers, health plans, and healthcare clearinghouses.

_____ 19. The freedom and ability to conduct one's life according to personal decisions, without external controls.

_____ 20. The appropriation of another person's ideas, processes, results, or words without giving appropriate credit.

EXERCISE 2: LINKING IDEAS

Directions: Fill in the blanks with the appropriate responses.

1. List the four elements of the research informed consent process.

   a. _____

   b. _____

   c. _____

   d. _____

2. Identify five general information requirements that are included in a comprehensive study consent form.

   a. _____

   b. _____

   c. _____

   d. _____

   e. _____

3. Study participants with _____ _____ (e.g., the mentally ill, cognitively impaired, or children) may be incompetent to consent to participate in research.

4. A study conducted by a student must be reviewed by their university faculty and also the _____ of the university and the agency where data will be collected.

5. The three levels of institutional review of research are:

   a. _____

   b. _____

   c. _____

6. Who determines the level of institutional review for a study? _____

   _____

7. During a presentation of study findings, a researcher inadvertently shows raw data, which includes subjects' names and Hepatitis C infection (yes or no) of the participants. This error is an example of a _____ _____. Provide a rationale for your answer. _____

   _____

   _____

   _____

   _____

8. A study that involved comparing the effects of an experimental medication on participants' serum lipid values to the effects of an existing medication on serum lipid values would probably require which type of institutional review? _____

9. Each federal agency that funds research with human participants has a chapter in the *Code of Federal Regulations* that protect the rights of the participants. Because of the similarities, these chapters as a group are called the _____.

10. Identify three possible types of research misconduct.

    a. _____

    b. _____

    c. _____

11. Is research misconduct present in nursing? (**Yes** or **No**) Provide a rationale for your answer.

    _____

    _____

    _____

    _____

    _____

Historical Events, Ethical Codes, and Regulations

Directions: Match each unethical study listed below with the correct description. You will use all answers more than once. The term subjects is deliberately used in these answers because the rights of the study participants were violated.

Unethical Study
 a. Tuskegee Syphilis Study
 b. Nazi Medical Experiments
 c. Jewish Chronic Disease Hospital Study
 d. Willowbrook Study

Description

_____ 1. Subjects were exposed to freezing temperatures, high altitudes, poisons, untested drugs, infections and surgeries without anesthesia.

_____ 2. The study was conducted to determine the natural course of syphilis in Black men.

_____ 3. Subjects were deliberately infected with Hepatitis A virus in this study.

_____ 4. Subjects and physicians providing care for the subjects were unaware that the study was being conducted.

_____ 5. Subjects did not receive penicillin when it was identified during the course of the study as an effective treatment for their disease.

_____ 6. The purpose of this study was to determine the patients' rejection responses to live cancer cells.

_____ 7. The subjects in this study were institutionalized children with mental disabilities.

_____ 8. The Nuremberg Code was developed in response to these unethical experiments.

_____   9. Subjects commonly sustained permanent physical damage or were killed.

_____   10. The National Commission for the Protection of Human Subjects of Biomedical and Behavioral Research, which wrote the Belmont Report, was formed in response to the public outcry over this study.

Federal Regulations Influencing the Conduct of Research

Directions: Match the federal regulation with the content or definitions provided. You will use some answers more than once. Review Table 4.1 for a summary of these regulations.

Federal Regulation
a. Health Insurance Portability and Accountability Act (HIPAA)
b. US Department of Health and Human Services (DHHS) Protection of Human Subjects Regulations (Common Rule)
c. US Food and Drug Administration (FDA) Protection of Human Subjects Regulations

Content or Definition

_____   1. Regulations provide direction for conducting research with participants vulnerable to coercion such as children and persons living in poverty or incarceration.

_____   2. Regulations were developed to protect identifiable private information (IPI).

_____   3. Regulations were originally developed in response to the Belmont Report and are part of the *Code of Federal Regulations* (CFR).

_____   4. Regulations are focused on clinical trials to test new drugs and medical devices.

_____   5. Regulations that apply to broader situations than research of human subjects.

Ethics of Published Studies

Directions: Match each ethical term to the appropriate example from the published studies provided in the appendices. You will use each answer only one time.

Ethical Term
a. Confidentiality
b. Coercion
c. Institutional review board (IRB)
d. Pseudonyms

Examples of Ethical Content From Published Studies

_____   1. The Steffen et al. (2021) study was conducted in Brazil (Appendix A). "The study began after submission to and approval by the Research Ethics Committee" (Steffen et al., 2021, p. e206). This approval is similar to approval that researchers would seek in the US from an _____ _____.

_____   2. Colwill et al. (2021) provided the demographic characteristics of the participants in Table 1 (Appendix B). To protect the confidentiality of the participants, they were identified in the table using _____.

_____ 3. The mixed methods study conducted by Greene and Ramos (2021) involved persons who had completed the Health Reform Monitoring Survey (HRMS) and indicated they were willing to be contacted for a follow up telephone interview (Appendix C). By only contacting potential participants who had given permission in advance for a follow up interview, the researchers implemented a safeguard against _____.

_____ 4. Greene and Ramos (2021, p. 1223) indicated that "identifying information was not retained nor connected to the transcripts or audio files." The lack of identifying information protected the _____ of the participants.

EXERCISE 3: WEB-BASED INFORMATION AND RESOURCES

Directions: Fill in the blanks with the appropriate websites.

1. Identify the website for the US Department of Health and Human Services (US DHHS, 2018) Code of Federal Regulations (45 CFR 46) for the protection of human subjects in research, which is also referred to as the "Common Rule."

_____

2. On this site, review Subpart B of 45 CFR 46. What groups of potential research participants are covered by Subpart B?

_____

_____

3. The ethical principles of respect for persons, beneficence, and justice were developed as part of the Belmont Report that guided the development of the DHHS regulations for the protection of human subjects in research. Locate the Belmont Report online:

_____

Using the copy of the Belmont Report that you found, answer Questions 4, 5, and 6.

4. When was the National Research Act (Pub. L. 93-348) signed into law?

_____

5. How many physicians were on the National Commission for the Protection of Human Subjects of Biomedical and Behavioral Research?

_____

How many nurses? _____

6. In Part C of the Belmont Report, respect for persons is linked to informed consent. Informed consent is further described as including what three major elements?

_____

_____

7. Identify the website for the Office of Research Integrity (ORI).

   _____

8. Find the Research Misconduct Case Summaries for 2021 on the ORI website. Provide an example with the researcher's last name and the type of misconduct.

   _____

   _____

9. Identify the website for Human Subjects Research at the National Human Genome Research Institute.

   _____

10. On the U.S. Food and Drug Administration (FDA) website, identify the special topic page on Clinical Trials and Human Subjects Protection.

    _____

EXERCISE 4: CONDUCTING CRITICAL APPRAISALS TO BUILD AN EVIDENCE-BASED PRACTICE

Directions: Chapter 4 in Grove and Gray (2023) has three sets of critical appraisal guidelines, with the final one being the guidelines to appraise the overall ethical aspects of the study. Use those guidelines and the research articles in Appendices A, B, and C to answer the following questions.

1. Describe the overall ethical aspects of the Steffen et al. (2021) article (Appendix A).

   _____

   _____

   _____

   _____

   _____

   _____

   _____

   _____

   _____

   _____

   _____

2. Describe the overall ethical aspects of the Colwill et al. (2021) article (Appendix B).

_____

_____

_____

_____

_____

_____

_____

_____

_____

_____

_____

3. Describe the overall ethical aspects of the Greene and Ramos (2021) article (Appendix C).

_____

_____

_____

_____

_____

_____

_____

_____

_____

_____

_____

_____

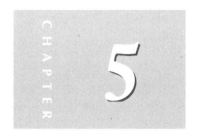

5 Examining Research Problems, Purposes, and Hypotheses

INTRODUCTION

You need to read Chapter 5 and then complete the following exercises. These exercises will assist you in critically appraising problems, purposes, objectives, questions, hypotheses, variables, and concepts in published studies. The answers to these exercises are in the Answer Key at the back of the book.

EXERCISE 1: TERMS AND DEFINITIONS

Directions: Match each term below with its correct definition. Each term is used only once and all terms are defined.

Terms

a. Conceptual definition
b. Demographic variables
c. Dependent variable
d. Extraneous variables
e. Hypothesis
f. Independent variable
g. Operational definition
h. Research problem
i. Research purpose
j. Research question
k. Research topic

Definitions

_____ 1. Description of how variables will be measured in a study, such as measuring acute pain in children with the FACES scale.

_____ 2. Clear, concise statement of the specific goal or focus of a study that is generated from the research problem.

_____ 3. The intervention or treatment that is manipulated or varied by the researcher to create an effect on the outcome variable.

_____ 4. Researchers attempt to identify and control the influence of these variables in quasi-experimental and experimental studies to reduce the potential for error in study findings.

_____ 5. Clear interrogative statement developed to direct a study, such as exploration of concepts in qualitative studies or determination of differences among groups in quantitative studies.

_____ 6. Variables reported in a study to describe the attributes or characteristics of study participants in the sample.

_____ 7. Formal statement of the expected relationship or outcome from studying variables in a specified population.

_____ 8. Concept or broad problem area, such as self-care, provides the basis for generating numerous research problems.

_____ 9. Definition that provides a variable or concept with theoretical meaning that could be obtained from a theory, concept analysis, or qualitative studies.

_____ 10. Area of concern or gap in nursing knowledge that requires research.

_____ 11. The response, behavior, or outcome predicted or explained in research; changes in this variable are presumed to be caused by the independent variable.

Types of Hypotheses

Directions: Match each type of hypothesis with the correct definition.

Type of Hypothesis

a. Associative hypothesis
b. Causal hypothesis
c. Complex hypothesis
d. Directional hypothesis
e. Nondirectional hypothesis
f. Null hypothesis
g. Research hypothesis
h. Simple hypothesis

Definitions

_____ 1. Hypothesis stating that no relationships exist among the variables studied.

_____ 2. Hypothesis stating that a relationship exists but not predicting the exact nature of the relationship.

_____ 3. Hypothesis stating the relationship (associative or causal) between two variables.

_____ 4. Hypothesis stating the specific nature of the interaction or relationship among two or more variables.

_____ 5. Hypothesis stating a relationship between two variables in which one variable (independent variable) is thought to cause or determine the presence of the other variable (dependent variable).

_____ 6. Hypothesis predicting the relationships (associative or causal) among three or more variables.

_____ 7. Alternative hypothesis to the null hypothesis; states that a relationship exists among two or more variables.

_____ 8. Hypothesis stating a relationship in which variables that occur or exist together in the real world is identified; thus when one variable changes, the other variables change.

EXERCISE 2: LINKING IDEAS

Research Problem and Purpose

Directions: Fill in the blanks with the appropriate responses.

1. A clearly stated research purpose includes:

   a. _____,

   b. _____, and usually the

   c. _____.

2. Research problems and purposes are significant if they have the potential to generate and refine relevant knowledge that:

   a. _____

   b. _____

   c. _____

3. The feasibility of a research problem and purpose is determined by examining the following:

   a. _____

   b. _____

   c. _____

   d. _____

4. Identify two national organizations or agencies that have developed lists of research priorities relevant to nursing.

   a. _____

   b. _____

5. When a study is funded by the National Institute of Nursing Research (NINR), the reader can know that the study is _____.

6. The purpose statement of qualitative studies usually includes _____, _____, and sometimes the setting.

7. Mason et al. (2021, p. 10) stated the purpose of their study was "to understand immigrant parents' health information seeking across ethnically diverse groups of immigrants who settled in Edmonton, Alberta." This purpose reflects what type of study:

   _____

8. Hernandez et al. (2021, p. 6) stated "The purpose of this research was to examine the outcomes of an inter-professional education (IPE) workshop on safe patient handling and mobility (SPM) for persons of size." This purpose is most reflective of what type of study?

   _____

9. The Methods section of mixed methods research includes both a _____ and _____ aspect.

10. Wahl et al. (2021, p. 417) conducted a study to "investigate associations between selective demographic and clinical variables, psychological well-being, and health literacy" in patients with chronic obstructive pulmonary disease. This purpose reflects what type of study? _____

Understanding Hypotheses

Directions: Ten sample hypotheses are presented in this section. Identify each hypothesis using the terms listed below. Four terms are needed to identify each hypothesis (associative versus causal, complex versus simple, directional versus nondirection, and null versus research). The correct answer for hypothesis #1 is provided as an example.

Terms

a. Associative hypothesis
b. Causal hypothesis
c. Complex hypothesis
d. Simple hypothesis
e. Directional hypothesis
f. Nondirectional hypothesis
g. Null hypothesis
h. Research hypothesis

Hypotheses

<u>b, c, e, h</u>   1. Relaxation therapy is more effective than standard care in decreasing pain perception and use of pain medications in adults with chronic arthritic pain.

_____   2. Age, family support, and health status are related to the self-care abilities of nursing-home residents.

_____   3. People vaccinated for COVID-19 have fewer positive COVID tests, lower hospitalization rates, less days in intensive care, and fewer deaths.

_____   4. Quality of life is related to self-care abilities in adults with mental illness.

_____   5. Healthy adults involved in an exercise program have lower low-density lipoprotein (LDL), higher high-density lipoprotein (HDL), and lower cardiovascular risk levels than adults not involved in the program.

_____   6. Low-back massage is more effective in decreasing perception of low-back pain than no massage in patients with chronic low-back pain.

_____   7. There are no relationships among the variables child depression, child behavior problems, child substance use, and bullying in a sample of middle school children in grades 7 to 9.

_____   8. Increased time on the operating table, lower diastolic blood pressure, higher age, and lower preoperative albumin levels are related to the increased development of pressure ulcers in hospitalized older adults.

_____   9. Intensive care unit (ICU) patients exposed to an audio tape of a significant family member's voice have less delirium than ICU patients without exposure to an audio tape.

_____   10. Nurses assigned to care for patients with COVID perceive more work stress and fatigue and report fewer hours of sleep than nurses caring for other types of patients.

_____   11. Patients with Type 2 diabetes mellitus who were managed using a mobile app have no lower hemoglobin A1c than those receiving standard care in a clinic.

_____   12. Healthcare providers who listen closely to patients, treat them as individuals, and demonstrate competence are predicted to build strong trust with their patients.

_____   13. Overweight individuals receiving nurse counseling through a designated website lose more weight and exercise more minutes per week than those receiving standard education.

14. State hypothesis #2 as a directional hypothesis.

_____

_____

_____

15. State hypothesis #6 as a null hypothesis.

_____

_____

_____

Identifying Types of Study Variables

Directions: Match each example variable below with the most likely type of variable that might be included in a study. All the variable types will be used more than once.

Type of Variable
a. Demographic variable
b. Dependent variable
c. Independent variable

Example Variables

_____   1. Age

_____   2. COVID immunization plan provided by text messaging

_____   3. Perception of pain

_____   4. Gender

_____   5. Length of hospital stay

_____   6. Race/Ethnic background

_____ 7. Bone density value

_____ 8. Educational level

_____ 9. Low-back massage

_____ 10. Depression level

_____ 11. Yoga classes

_____ 12. Hemoglobin A1c

_____ 13. Low-density lipoprotein (LDL) value

_____ 14. Body mass index (BMI)

_____ 15. DVD on nutrition presented in clinic

Understanding Study Variables

Directions: Match these variables with the examples provided below. Some of the variables will be used more than once.

Terms
a. Demographic variables
b. Dependent variables
c. Extraneous variable
d. Independent variable
e. Research concept

Examples

_____ 1. Acute pain is a physiological and psychological response to trauma that is commonly examined in studies.

_____ 2. When researchers examined the effects of nasal oxygen on oral temperature, all patients with fever were excluded from the study because fever had the potential to affect the study's findings. This is an example of what type of variable?

_____ 3. Six-week physical therapy program for the elderly over 70 years of age.

_____ 4. Variables such as age, gender, and medical diagnoses are measured to describe the sample.

_____ 5. Understanding bullying experienced by school aged children.

_____ 6. Type 2 diabetes mellitus (T2DM) educational program provided through a mobile application on the patients' phone.

_____ 7. Family income of participants

_____ 8. Introduction of a shelter cat into the homes of children with ASD [Autism Spectrum Disorder]

_____ 9. Temperature, oxygen saturation, pulse, and blood pressure of patients with COVID-19

_____ 10. Implementing a trust exercise with patients facing a terminal diagnosis.

EXERCISE 3: WEB-BASED INFORMATION AND RESOURCES

Directions: The following questions require identifying and searching selected websites. Review the key information provided on the websites.

1. The Centers for Disease Control and Prevention (CDC) report statistical information that is useful in documenting the significance of a research problem. Identify the home page for the CDC:

   _____

2. On the CDC website, search for the topic: "Violence Prevention." Did you find information about child abuse and neglect prevention? (**Yes** or **No**) Identify the website for this topic:

   _____

   _____

3. Identify the CDC website that provides resources related to overweight and obesity.

   _____

4. Identify the CDC website that provides information about coronavirus vaccines for you and your patients.

   _____

5. The Oncology Nursing Society (ONS) website includes a variety of resources for nurses. What is the website for ONS?

   _____

6. Identify the website for the National Institute of Nursing Research (NINR):

   _____

   _____

7. Identify the website for the NINR Mission and Strategic Plan. This document will help you determine if a study is significant to NINR and a focus of funding.

   _____

   _____

8. Identify the website for the American Diabetes Association so you read more about the management of Type2DM.

   _____

EXERCISE 4: CONDUCTING CRITICAL APPRAISALS TO BUILD AN EVIDENCE-BASED PRACTICE

Problem and Purpose

Steffen et al. (2021) Study

Directions: Review the Steffen et al. (2021) research article in Appendix A and answer the following questions.

1. State the problem of this study.

    a. Significance: _____

    _____

    _____

    _____

    _____

    _____

    b. Background: _____

    _____

    _____

    _____

    _____

    _____

    c. What was the problem statement reported in the Steffen et al. (2021) study?

    _____

    _____

    _____

    _____

2. State the purpose of this study. _____

    _____

    _____

    _____

3. Are the problem and the purpose significant? (**Yes** or **No**) Provide a rationale for your answer.

_____

_____

_____

_____

_____

_____

4. Review the research purpose in the Steffen et al. (2021) study and determine if the variables, population, and setting were identified. Then address the following questions.

   a. Identify the variables. _____

   _____

   _____

   _____

   b. Identify the population. _____

   c. Identify the setting. _____

5. Is it feasible for Steffen et al. (2021) to study the problem and purpose? (**Yes** or **No**) Provide a rationale.

_____

_____

_____

_____

_____

_____

_____

Colwill et al. (2021) Study

Directions: Review the Colwill et al. (2021) research article in Appendix B and answer the following questions.

1. State the problem of this study.

    a. Significance: _____

    _____

    _____

    _____

    _____

    _____

    _____

    b. Background: _____

    _____

    _____

    _____

    _____

    _____

    c. Problem statement: _____

    _____

    _____

    _____

    _____

2. Study purpose

    a. What was the purpose of this study? _____

    _____

    _____

b. What did the authors state that provided the best direction for their study? Include this content.

_____

_____

_____

_____

c. State a clear purpose that could be used to direct this study: _____

_____

_____

3. Are the problem and purpose significant? (**Yes** or **No**) Provide a rationale.

_____

_____

_____

_____

_____

4. Did the purpose identified the concepts, population, and setting for this study?

a. Identify the research concepts. _____

_____

b. Identify the population. _____

c. Identify the setting. _____

5. What factors made studying this problem and purpose feasible for these researchers?

_____

_____

_____

_____

_____

_____

Greene and Ramos (2021) Study

Directions: Review the Greene and Ramos (2021) research article in Appendix C and answer the following questions.

1. State the problem of this study.

    a. Significance: _____

    _____

    _____

    _____

    _____

    b. Background: _____

    _____

    _____

    _____

    _____

    _____

    _____

    _____

    c. Problem statement: _____

    _____

    _____

    _____

2. a. State the purpose for the Greene and Ramos (2021) study. _____

    _____

    _____

    b. Was the purpose clear and concise in this study? (**Yes** or **No**) Provide a rationale for your answer.

    _____

    _____

    _____

    _____

3. Are the problem and the purpose significant? (**Yes** or **No**) Provide a rationale. _____

    _____

    _____

    _____

    _____

    _____

    _____

4. Does the purpose identify the concepts and/or variables, population, and setting for this study? _____

    _____

    a. Identify the research concepts and/or variables. _____

        _____

        _____

        _____

    b. Identify the population(s). _____

        _____

    c. Identify the setting(s). _____

        _____

5. Is it feasible for these researchers to study this problem and purpose? (**Yes** or **No**) Provide a rationale.

    _____

    _____

    _____

    _____

    _____

    _____

Objectives, Questions, and Hypotheses

Steffen et al. (2021) Study

Directions: Review this study in Appendix A and answer the following questions.

1. Are objectives, questions, or hypotheses stated in this study? Identify them. _____

    _____

    _____

2. Are they appropriate and clearly stated? (**Yes** or **No**) Provide a rationale for your answer. _____

    _____

    _____

    _____

    _____

    _____

Colwill et al. (2021) Study

Directions: Review this study in Appendix B and answer the following questions.

1. Are objectives, questions, or hypotheses stated in this study? Identify them. _____

    _____

    _____

    _____

2. Are they appropriate and clearly stated? (**Yes** or **No**) Provide a rationale for your answer. _____

    _____

    _____

    _____

    _____

Greene and Ramos (2021) Study

***Directions:* Review this study in Appendix C and answer the following questions.**

1. Are objectives, questions, or hypotheses stated in this study? Identify them. _____

   _____

   _____

   _____

   _____

   _____

2. Are they appropriate and clearly stated for a mixed methods study? Provide a rationale for your answer.

   _____

   _____

   _____

   _____

Research Variables or Concepts*

Steffen et al. (2021) Study

Directions: Review this study in Appendix A and answer the following questions.

1. List the major variables in this study and identify the type of each variable (independent, dependent, or research).

Variable	Type of variable

---

*Colwill et al. (2021) study research concepts are discussed and critically appraised in more detail in Chapter 3 Introduction to Qualitative Research of this study guide.

2. Identify the conceptual and operational definitions for the MI intervention.

   a. Conceptual definition: _____

   _____

   _____

   _____

   _____

   _____

   b. Operational definition: _____

   _____

   _____

   _____

   _____

3. Are these definitions clear? (**Yes** or **No**) Provide a rationale for your answer.

   _____

   _____

   _____

   _____

   _____

4. Identify the demographic variables in the study.

   _____

   _____

   _____

   _____

5. Identify the extraneous variables measured in this study. What was the rationale for measuring these?

Variables: _____

Rationale: _____

_____

_____

_____

_____

Greene and Ramos (2021) Study

Directions: Review this study in Appendix C and answer the following questions.

1. List the research concept in the qualitative part of this study.

_____

_____

2. Identify the demographic variables in the study. _____

_____

_____

_____

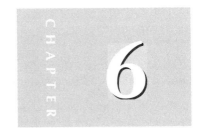

6 Understanding and Critically Appraising the Literature Review

INTRODUCTION

After reading Chapter 6, complete the following exercises. These exercises will assist you in reading and critically appraising the literature reviews in research reports. The answers for the following exercises are in the Answer Key at the back of the book.

EXERCISE 1: TERMS AND DEFINITIONS

Directions: Match each term below with its correct definition. Each term is used only once and all terms are defined.

Terms

a. Article
b. Bibliographic database
c. Citation
d. Clinical journals
e. Conference proceedings
f. Data-based literature
g. Landmark studies
h. Peer reviewed

i. Primary source
j. Reference
k. Relevant studies
l. Replication studies
m. Secondary source
n. Textbook
o. Theoretical literature
p. Thesis

Definitions

_____ 1. Reproductions of a study undertaken to determine if the results are the same in different settings or with different samples.

_____ 2. A paper about a specific topic published together with similar documents on similar themes in journals, encyclopedias, or edited books.

_____ 3. Source, whose author summarizes or quotes content from a primary source.

_____ 4. Literature that includes concept analyses, conceptual maps, theories, and conceptual frameworks that support a selected research problem and purpose.

_____ 5. Papers that were evaluated by other scholars as being of high quality, trustworthy, and acceptable for publication.

_____ 6. Source, whose author originated or is responsible for generating the ideas published.

_____ 7. Paraphrasing or quoting content from a source, using it as an example, or presenting it as support for a position taken.

_____ 8. Periodicals that include research reports and non-research articles about professional issues and practice problems.

_____ 9. Research that has a direct bearing on the study being planned or topic of concern.

_____ 10. The author, year, title of a source, and publication information that allows a reader to find the publication to which the author is referring.

_____ 11. Compilations of citations and references that are searchable and allow the researcher to find articles and other publications on a specific topic.

_____ 12. A research project completed by a student as part of the requirements for a master's degree.

_____ 13. Research reports that are published in journals, books, dissertations, and theses.

_____ 14. Compilations of abstracts and papers presented at a professional meeting that may include the findings of pilot studies and preliminary studies.

_____ 15. Significant research projects that influenced a discipline and led to the development of additional studies on the topic.

_____ 16. A source with multiple chapters written to provide content related to a course taught by instructors in an education setting.

EXERCISE 2: LINKING IDEAS

Examples of Main Ideas From the Chapter

Directions: Fill in the blanks with the appropriate word(s)/response(s).

1. The process of reviewing the literature has four components, which are (1) finding _____ research reports and theoretical sources; (2) _____ _____ the sources; (3) _____ the results; and (4) developing an _____ and _____ reference list.

2. The review of the literature identifies what is _____ and what is _____ _____ about a specific topic.

3. A high-quality review of literature contains both _____ and _____ knowledge about a specific topic.

4. Current sources for a literature review are defined as those that were published within _____ years of when the article was accepted for publication.

5. Unlike qualitative studies where the timing and depth of a literature review may vary, the literature review is consistently conducted at the beginning of the research process to direct the planning and implementing of a(n) _____ study.

6. A _____ is a journal that is published over time and is numbered sequentially for the years published.

7. A _____-_____ article means that the paper was selected for publication based on the input of scholars who were experts in the paper's topic.

8. A well-written summary of a review of the literature provides direction for the formation of the _____ of the study.

9. Although information is readily available online, not all of the information websites provide is _____, _____, and/or _____.

10. A literature _____ _____ or _____ _____ can be used to help process the information from numerous studies and identify the key aspects of the study (authors, year, purpose, design, sample, measurement methods, and results).

Theoretical and Empirical Sources

Directions: Theoretical and empirical sources are included in the literature review of a published study. Review the references below and label each with a **T** if it is a theoretical source or an **E** if it is an empirical source. The final determination of the type of source would be made by reviewing the source.

_____ 1. Watson, J. (2012). *Human caring science: A theory of nursing* (2nd ed.). Jones & Bartlett.

_____ 2. Abstracts from the Western Institute of Nursing Research Conference.

_____ 3. Master's thesis comparing acute pain of persons with neuropathy to the acute pain of persons post abdominal surgery.

_____ 4. Reuben, M., Mohamed, F., & Mutasa, F. (2021). Strategies for preventing and responding to sexual violence against children in Rombo District, Tanzania: A mixed methods study. *Open Journal of Social Science, 9*(9). 439–453. https://doi.org/10.4236/jss.2021.99032

_____ 5. Yip, J. (2021). Theory-based advanced nursing practice: A practice update on the application of Orem's Self-Care Deficit Nursing Theory. *SAGE Open Nursing, 7,* 1–7. https://doi.org/10.1177/23779608211011993

_____ 6. Lulgjuraj, D., Hubner, T., Radzinski, N., & Hopkins, U. (2021). Everyone is someone's child: The experiences of pediatric nurses caring for adult COVID-19 patients. *Journal of Pediatric Nursing, 60,* 198–206. https://doi.org/10.1016/j.pedn.2021.06.015

_____ 7. Roy, C., & Andrews, H. (2008). *Roy Adaptation Model* (3rd ed.). Pearson.

_____ 8. Doctoral dissertation

_____ 9. von Bertalanffy, L. (2015). *General systems theory: Foundations, development, applications* (Revised ed.). Braziller.

_____ 10. Lim, H., & Yi, Y. (2021). Effects of a web-based education program for nurses using medical malpractice cases: A randomized control trial. *Nurse Education Today, 104.* Article 104997. https://doi.org/10.1016/j.nedt.2021.104997

Primary and Secondary Sources

Directions: A literature review includes mainly primary sources. Remember that a primary source is developed by the person conducting the research or developing the theory. A secondary source is the synthesis of primary and other sources. Based on these definitions, determine if a source is primary or secondary. Label each source below with a **P** if it is a primary source or an **S** if it is a secondary source.

_____   1.   Compilation and comparison of theories of adaptation

_____   2.   Doctoral dissertation

_____   3.   Roy, C., & Andrews, H. (2008). *Roy Adaptation Model* (3rd ed.). Pearson.

_____   4.   Review of studies to develop an evidence-based practice guideline

_____   5.   Seminal study comparing interventions for stress

_____   6.   Study published in *Applied Nursing Research*

_____   7.   Report of a pilot study to test the feasibility of an intervention

_____   8.   Published review of research textbook

_____   9.   Exact replication of a study

_____   10.   Phenomenological research article in *Journal of Nursing Scholarship*

EXERCISE 3: WEB-BASED INFORMATION AND RESOURCES

1.   Find the URL for an article published by Leite, Padilha, and Cecatti (2019) in the journal, *Clinics*, about writing a literature review.

_____

Use the article to answer question 2.

2.   What are the <u>five</u> steps of a literature review according to Leite et al. (2019)?

a. _____

b. _____

c. _____

d. _____

e. _____

3.   Find the National Institutes of Health (NIH) National Medical Library online.

_____

4. On the NIH National Medical Library site, find the section *Resources for You*. Then click on the resources For Health Professionals.

   _____

5. Find the website for the National Medical Library Catalog.

   _____

6. Purdue University has an Online Writing Library (OWL) that provides correct information about how to cite a source in American Psychology Association (APA) format. Find the website for OWL.

   _____

7. On the OWL website found in the previous question, find the information about how to write a literature review. What are the three parts of a written literature review?

   a. _____

   b. _____

   c. _____

8. The OWL article about writing a literature review describes four ways to organize a literature review. Select one of these ways and describe it in your own words.

   _____

   _____

   _____

   _____

9. Which of these four ways for organizing the literature review was used by Al-Shamaly (2021) in the article's Background section?
   Al-Shamaly, H. S. (2021). A focused ethnography of the culture of inclusive caring practice in the intensive care unit. *Nursing Open, 8,* 2973–2985. https://doi.org/10.1002/nop2.1009

   _____

   _____

   _____

   _____

EXERCISE 4: CONDUCTING CRITICAL APPRAISALS TO BUILD AN EVIDENCE-BASED PRACTICE

Directions: Review the three articles in Appendices A, B, and C to answer these questions. Use the critical appraisal guidelines in Chapter 6 of Grove and Gray (2023) to provide additional information.

Review the Introduction section and the Limitations section of the Steffen et al. (2021) article (Appendix A) to answer the following questions.

1. What are the main ideas of the three paragraphs of the Introduction?

_____

_____

_____

_____

2. Which citation in the Introduction referred to a meta-analysis of studies about nursing interventions for diabetes case management ?

_____

3. In the Limitations section, Steffen et al. (2021) cited three sources. Identify the authors and the type of reference of each source.

_____

_____

_____

_____

In the Colwill et al. (2021) article (Appendix B), use the reference list to answer the following 5 questions.

1. Were the references current? Provide your rationale using the number and percentage of the references published in the past 5 years and the past 10 years.

_____

_____

_____

2. Describe the two references that were older than 10 years. _____

_____

_____

_____

3. How many of the references were published in nursing journals? _____

4. Most of the references were published in journals for which profession?

   _____

   _____

   Why do you think they used these references instead of references in nursing journals?

   _____

   _____

5. Describe your evaluation of the quality and relevance of the references cited by Colwill et al. (2021).

   _____

   _____

   _____

   _____

   _____

Refer to the reference list of the Greene and Ramos (2021) article (Appendix C) to answer the following 5 questions.

1. Were the references current? Provide your rationale using the number and percentage of the references published in the past 5 years and the past 10 years. _____

   _____

   _____

2. Review the references that were older than 10 years. Identify one that described a measurement (scale or assessment) of patients' trust in their physician or provider.

   _____

3. Mechanic and Minor (2000) described which relevant concept of the study?

   _____

Read the Introduction section of the Greene and Ramos (2021) article to answer the remaining questions.

4. Were the studies cited in the Introduction critically appraised? Were they synthesized?

_____

_____

_____

_____

5. Was a concise summary provided in the Introduction? Did the researchers identify what was known and what was not known about trusting one's provider? Provide a rationale for your answer.

_____

_____

_____

_____

_____

_____

_____

_____

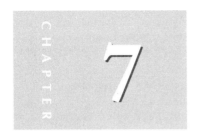

Understanding Theory and Research Frameworks

INTRODUCTION

You need to read Chapter 7 and then complete the following exercises. These exercises will assist you in learning key terms and identifying and critically appraising frameworks in published studies. The answers for the following exercises are in the Answer Key at the back of the book.

EXERCISE 1: TERMS AND DEFINITIONS

Directions: Match each term below with its correct definition. Each term is used only once and all terms are defined.

Terms

a. Abstract
b. Assumptions
c. Concept
d. Concrete
e. Construct
f. Middle range theory
g. Phenomena

h. Philosophies
i. Proposition
j. Research framework
k. Statement
l. Theory
m. Variables

Definitions

_____ 1. An abstract, logical structure of concepts that guides the development of the study and links the study findings to nursing's body of knowledge.

_____ 2. Rational intellectual explorations of truths or principles of being, knowledge, or conduct that influence theory development.

_____ 3. A broader category of ideas that may encompass several concepts.

_____ 4. Statements that are considered true without testing, such as patients want to increase their self-care.

_____ 5. The component of a theory that describes type of relationship that exists between or among concepts.

_____ 6. A term that abstractly names an object or phenomenon.

_____ 7. A statement that describes the relationships among two or more concepts.

_____ 8. Thinking oriented towards the development of a general idea, without association with a particular instance.

_____ 9. Theories that are less abstract than grand theories; focus on patients' health conditions, family situations, and nursing actions; and are often tested in quantitative research.

_____ 10. The conscious awareness of an experience that may be described by a concept, statement, or theory.

_____ 11. A set of concepts and statements that present a view of a phenomenon.

_____ 12. Concepts that have been operationally defined so that they can be measured.

_____ 13. Thinking oriented toward a particular instance; often can be observed or felt.

Types of Theories

Directions: Match each type of theory below with its correct definition. Each term is used only once and all terms are defined.

Terms
a. Grand nursing theory
b. Implicit frameworks
c. Scientific theory
d. Situation-specific theory
e. Substantive theory
f. Tentative theory

_____ 1. A middle range theory that is narrower in focus; limited to a specific population, phenomenon, or specialty.

_____ 2. Abstract theories that are labeled as conceptual models or conceptual frameworks by some scholars.

_____ 3. Underdeveloped theoretical ideas that may come from the linkages among variables found in other studies that are used to guide a study but are not clearly developed into a research framework.

_____ 4. A newly proposed framework synthesized from the findings of other studies or multiple theories.

_____ 5. Theories of genetics or pathophysiology that are supported by extensive research evidence and whose relational statements may be called _laws_.

_____ 6. Another name for a middle range theory; the theory is more concrete and applicable to the substance of clinical practice.

EXERCISE 2: LINKING IDEAS

Key Theoretical Ideas

Directions: Fill in the blanks with the appropriate word(s)/response(s).

1. The elements of theory are concepts and _____ about the relationships among the concepts.

2. A(n) _____, such as perceived pain, is less abstract than a concept and is defined so that it is measurable in a study.

3. The _____ of a theory are tested through research.

4. Statements at the lowest level of abstraction that are identified in a quantitative study to be tested are referred to as _____.

5. The Self-Care Deficit Theory of Nursing was written by _____.

6. Covell (2008) published a middle range theory of _____.

7. _____ _____ are the theoretical concepts and statements that guide the development of a study and allows the researcher to link the findings back to nursing's body of knowledge.

8. How are the conceptual definition and operational definition of a variable different?

   _____

   _____

   _____

   _____

   _____

   _____

9. How are grand nursing theories and middle range theories different? Provide an example of each type of theory.

   _____

   _____

   _____

   _____

   _____

   _____

10. How are scientific theories and tentative theories different?

   _____

   _____

   _____

   _____

   _____

   _____

Levels of Abstraction

Directions: Place the following terms in order from the highest level of abstraction to the lowest level of abstraction.

Variable (example – Social Support Score)
Construct (example – Holistic Response to Life Stressors)
Operational definition (Participant's total score on the Social Support Scale, comprised of 20 items with a 1 to 5 Likert scale)
Concept (example-Perceived social support)

_____ *(highest level of abstraction)*

_____

_____

_____ *(lowest level of abstraction)*

Elements of Theory

Directions: Study the diagram below and answer the following questions in the spaces provided.

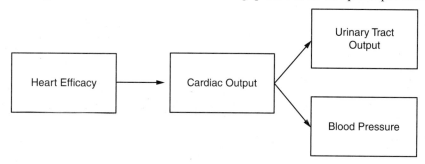

1. List the concepts in the diagram.

    _____

    _____

2. What do the arrows represent?

    _____

    _____

3. What does this figure represent when included in a study?

    _____

Examples of Frameworks

Directions: Several theories were identified in Chapter 7 that had been used in nursing studies. Match the statement about the theory to the appropriate theorist's name by using the focus of the middle range theories in Table 7.4 in your textbook, *Understanding Nursing Research*, 8th edition.

Theorist(s)

a. Byrne et al.
b. Kolcaba
c. Lenz et al.
d. Mishel
e. Meleis
f. Reed
g. Riegel et al.
h. Swanson

Middle Range Theory

_____ 1. The caring aspects of the nurse–patient relationships promote well-being.

_____ 2. Comfort is an immediate desirable outcome of nurses' interventions.

_____ 3. Consistent with Orem's theory, a person living with a chronic disease time must develop knowledge and care for themselves.

_____ 4. Nurses are often with persons who are experiencing transitions, changes in their life situations that may affect their health.

_____ 5. The interaction of multiple symptoms adds to the complexity of living with illness.

_____ 6. Persons facing life-threatening events may acquire an expanded view of self and the environment, a perspective that has been labeled self-transcendence.

_____ 7. When facing a new diagnosis, people may experience uncertainty because they do not understand the meaning of the illness-related events and cannot accurately predict the outcome.

_____ 8. Surgeons, nurses, and others in the operating room wearing personal protective equipment experience occupational stress because of becoming hot.

Example of Grand Nursing Theory Used in a Study

Directions: In Chapter 7, find the discussion about the study by Lok et al. (2021) and answer the following questions.

1. Which grand nursing theory was used as the framework for this study?

_____

2. From the research excerpt and the critical appraisal, identify the application of Roy's concept to the study.

a. Focal stimulus _____

b. Degree of coping and adaptation _____

c. Nursing action to promote adaptation _____

3. What was the instrument used to measure the person's response to CST? _____

_____

EXERCISE 3: WEB-BASED INFORMATION AND RESOURCES

Directions: Provide the appropriate responses for the following questions in the spaces provided.

1. Identify a website that describes Kolcaba's middle range theory of comfort.

   _____

2. Using the website you identified, what are Kolcaba's three types of comfort? She identified these in 1991.

   a. _____

   b. _____

   c. _____

3. Select one of the theories on Table 7.4, other than Kolcaba's comfort theory, and find a website with additional information about the theory. You will use the website or article to answer the next question. List the website you found here:

   _____

4. On the website about the middle range theory you selected, identify 3 concepts of the theory.

   _____

   _____

EXERCISE 4: CONDUCTING CRITICAL APPRAISALS TO BUILD AN EVIDENCE-BASED PRACTICE

Directions: Read and conduct critical appraisals of the framework or theoretical sections of the following research reports.

Steffen et al. (2021) Critical Appraisal

Review the Steffen et al. (2021) study to answer the following questions. The article is at the back of the study guide as Appendix A.

1. Steffen et al. (2021) identified the Chronic Care Model as the basis for the risk strata. What two concepts from the theory do they identify?

   _____

   _____

2. How were the risk strata used in the study?

   _____

   _____

   _____

3. The source cited by the authors for the Chronic Care Model is a non-English language reference. Because of that, search the Institute for Healthcare Improvement website for a diagram showing the elements of the Chronic Care Model. Provide the URL here:

    _____

4. Using the diagram, identify three concepts (phrases or terms) included in the model.

    _____

    _____

    _____

5. How might the researchers have linked the intervention, the nurses who implemented the intervention, and the study outcomes to the concepts in the model? Doing this would have made the research framework more explicit.

    _____

    _____

    _____

    _____

6. How might the researchers have improved the integration of the model into the study?

    _____

    _____

    _____

    _____

Colwill et al. (2021) Critical Appraisal

Review the Colwill et al. (2021) to answer the following questions. The article is provided as Appendix B.

1. Colwill et al. (2021) developed a model from their analysis of the interview data. Identify the 5 concepts that are displayed in the outer ring representing the construct of society.

    _____

    _____

2. The person is another construct in the model. What are the three concepts drawn around the person to represent processes?

_____

_____

3. Identify part of a participant quotation that supports one of the concepts around the person.

_____

_____

_____

_____

4. The person enters the healthcare system, the third construct in the model, because of the catalyst of endocarditis. What 3 additional concepts emerged?

_____

_____

5. What was the core concept identified by the researchers?

_____

6. In the last paragraph of 4. Discussion (prior to 4.1), the researchers mention transitions. To which existing middle-range theory could the researchers have linked their findings? If unsure, review Table 7.4 in Chapter 4 of the textbook. _____

7. What are the strengths of model developed by the researchers? What are the weaknesses?

_____

_____

_____

_____

Green and Ramos (2021) Critical Appraisal

1. Trust is a construct and the focus of the mixed methods study. Different ways that trust has been conceptually and operationally defined were included in the Introduction section. Identify a measurement method (operational definition) of trust used in previous studies.

    _____

    _____

2. For the operational definition you selected, write a conceptual definition, using information in the Introduction section.

    _____

    _____

    _____

3. From the researchers' analysis of the qualitative data, what key dimensions (concepts) of trust emerged? The dimensions are also displayed in Figure 1. Restate these concepts as a conceptual definition of trust.

    _____

    _____

    _____

4. Of the concepts identified in Figure 1 in the article, which one had the strongest relationship with trust?

    _____

5. Green and Ramos provided insights into better measures of patient trust in healthcare providers. What could they have done, however, to more effectively link their findings to theoretical literature?

    _____

    _____

    _____

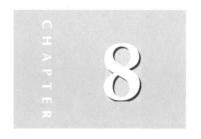

CHAPTER 8

Clarifying Quantitative Research Designs

INTRODUCTION

You need to read Chapter 8 and then complete the following exercises. These exercises will assist you in learning key terms, understanding design validity, and identifying and critically appraising quantitative research designs in published studies. The answers for these exercises are in the Answer Key at the back of the book.

EXERCISE 1: TERMS AND DEFINITIONS

Understanding Common Design Terms

Directions: Match each term below with its correct definition. Each term is used only once and all terms are defined.

Terms

a. Bias	j. Manipulation
b. Blinding	k. Multicausality
c. Causality	l. Noninterventional design
d. Control	m. Probability
e. Correlational design	n. Quasi-experimental design
f. Cross-sectional design	o. Randomized controlled trial (RCT)
g. Descriptive design	p. Research design
h. Experimental design	q. Retrospective
i. Longitudinal design	

Definitions

_____ 1. Implementing an intervention and ensuring it is being implemented consistently; form of control in interventional studies

_____ 2. Blueprint or detailed plan for conducting a study.

_____ 3. Distortion of study findings that are slanted or deviated from the true or expected.

_____ 4. Type of design that facilitates the search for knowledge and examination of causality in situations where control is limited in some ways.

_____ 5. Type of design that involves examining a group of study participants simultaneously in various stages of development, severity of illness, or levels of education to describe changes in a phenomenon over stages.

_____ 6. A study that looks back by using data that were previously collected.

_____ 7. The power to prevent unplanned changes in the environment, interventions, and other factors that might affect a study outcome. This is greater in experimental than quasi-experimental designs.

_____ 8. Study design that examines relationships between or among two or more variables in a single group.

_____ 9. A strategy that prevents participants from knowing whether they are in the treatment or comparison group; data collectors also may not know which participants are in each group.

_____ 10. The recognition that several interrelating variables can be involved in causing a particular outcome.

_____ 11. Descriptive and correlational designs are referred to as these types of designs since the focus is on examining variables as they naturally occur in the environment and not on the implementation of an intervention by researchers.

_____ 12. Research designs conducted to gain information about variables in relatively new areas of study, such as studies to identify problems in current practice, determine trends of illnesses, and categorize information.

_____ 13. Addresses relative rather than absolute causality.

_____ 14. Designs that involve collecting data from the same study participants at different points in time and might also be referred to as repeated measures.

_____ 15. Type of design focused on examining causality where extensive control of the intervention, setting, sampling process, and extraneous variables is possible.

_____ 16. Type of study conducted in nursing and medicine that is noted to be the strongest methodology for testing the effectiveness of an intervention due to the elements of design that limit the potential for bias. These studies are best conducted in multiple geographical locations to increase the sample size and obtain a more representative sample.

_____ 17. Examines the effect of a single intervention on a selected outcome.

Design Validity Terms

Directions: Match each term below with its correct definition. Each term is used only once and all terms are defined.

Types of Design Validity
a. Construct design validity
b. External design validity
c. Internal design validity
d. Statistical conclusion design validity

Definitions

_____ 1. Validity concerned with the extent to which study findings can be generalized beyond the sample used in the study.

_____ 2. Validity concerned with whether the decisions about relationships or differences drawn from statistical analysis are an accurate reflection of the real world

_____ 3. Validity concerned with the fit between the conceptual and operational definitions of the study variables and the quality of the measurement methods used in the study.

_____ 4. Validity concerned with whether the study findings are a true reflection of reality, rather than the result of extraneous variables.

Threats to Design Validity

a. Attrition
b. Experimenter expectancy
c. History
d. Inadequate definitions of variables
e. Interaction of sample and setting
f. Interaction of selection and intervention
g. Intervention fidelity

h. Low statistical power
i. Maturation
j. Mono-operation bias
k. Participant assignment to groups
l. Participant selection
m. Social desirability
n. Unreliable measurement methods

Definitions

_____ 1. Only one measurement method was used to measure a study variable.

_____ 2. Occurred when an event not related to the planned study happened during the study that could have an impact on the findings.

_____ 3. Variables were not being consistently measured during a study.

_____ 4. Participants became wiser or more tired over the course of a study.

_____ 5. Participants selected answers based on wanting the researcher to like them or based on behaviors that are perceived as positive.

_____ 6. Percentage of participants who withdrew from the study exceeded 25%.

_____ 7. Many potential participants declined to be in the study because the time and effort required by the intervention was too great.

_____ 8. Participants were placed in groups using non-random methods in an interventional study.

_____ 9. Theoretical or conceptual definitions did not clearly define the concepts to be measured.

_____ 10. The researchers' preferences and predictions biased or influenced the outcomes of a study.

_____ 11. The study intervention was not delivered consistently to all participants in the experimental group.

_____ 12. Concluding there was no difference between groups or no relationships when a difference or relationship exists.

_____ 13. Participants selected in a specific setting were unique and did not resemble the population

_____ 14. Participants who had unique characteristics were selected by nonrandom sampling methods.

EXERCISE 2: LINKING IDEAS

Directions: Fill in the blanks in this section with the appropriate word(s).

1. Studies with interventions such as quasi-experimental and experimental designs are implemented to examine _____.

2. Quasi-experimental and experimental studies include the manipulation of an independent variable that is called the study _____.

3. The purpose of quasi-experimental and experimental research designs is to maximize _____ of factors, such as extraneous variables, in the study situation.

4. Using a(n) _____ orientation, researchers design studies to examine the likelihood that a given effect will occur under a defined set of circumstances.

5. Interventional studies cannot be retrospective studies; they are _____ studies.

6. Critical appraisal of research involves being able to think through threats to _____ that occurred and make judgments about how seriously they affected the integrity of the study findings.

7. Hypothesis: Family history of cardiovascular disease (CVD), pack year history of smoking a pack a day for 5 or more years. obesity, lack of exercise, and untreated hypertension increase the likelihood of a myocardial infarction in adults. This hypothesis should be tested using a _____ _____ design.

8. In an experimental study, the study participants are randomly assigned to either the _____ group or the _____ group.

9. Developing a quality intervention and implementing it consistently in a study using a protocol promotes _____ in the study.

10. A researcher wants to add _____ to the design of a study by limiting the sample to only first-time mothers who are 40 or more years old.

11. The study was implemented using a _____ design to compare the differences between two existing group, such as the rate of missed appointments at Clinic A compared to the rate of missed appointments at Clinic B.

12. List three elements of quasi-experimental and experimental designs that are focused on examining causality.

    a. _____

    _____

    b. _____

    _____

    c. _____

    _____

13. No relationship was found between missed appointments and medication adherence in a study with 35 hypertension patients recruited from a practice of physicians and nurse practitioners. The researchers suggest that there may have been a Type II error. The Type II error was most likely due to? _____
_____

14. The longitudinal study began with a sample of 100 but only 70 of the participants completed the study. _____ was a threat to internal design validity.

15. The study had a sample of over 300 participants but the researchers noted that the primary instruments' internal reliability consistency was 0.62 using Cronbach's alpha. This represents a threat to _____ _____design validity.

Determining Types of Design Validity in Studies

Directions: Match the type of design validity with the examples provided from studies. The types of design validity may be used more than once. Use the listed tables in the textbook chapter to figure out the correct answers.

Types of Design Validity
a. Construct validity (Table 8.1, p. 209)
b. External validity (Table 8.4, p. 216)
c. Internal validity (Table 8.2, p. 211)
d. Statistical conclusion validity (Table 8.3, p. 214)

Study Examples

_____ 1. Over 40% of the potential study participants approached, declined to participate because they did not want to follow a structured low-calorie diet. This interaction of the selection of participants and the study intervention is an example of what type of threat to design validity?

_____ 2. A study had a sample of 623 adults over 70 years of age and statistically significant relationships were found among the variables of body mass index (BMI), cholesterol values, and hemoglobin Alc. This indicates which type of design validity?

_____ 3. The study report included a theoretical definition of depression that was consistent with the operational definition, which was the participants' scores on the Beck Depression Inventory. This is an indicator of which type of design validity?

_____ 4. The study participants were survivors of myocardial infarctions (MI) who were in cardiac rehabilitation (intervention group) compared to MI survivors who did not choose to participate in cardiac rehabilitation (comparison group). The hypothesis was that participation in cardiac rehabilitation reduces blood pressure values, increases resting oxygen levels, and lowers the frequency of angina one-year post-MI. The study methods indicated a threat to which type of design validity?

_____ 5. The findings of an interventional study conducted in three Magnet-designated hospitals were considered for application in a system of community hospitals that were not supportive of research. Prior to application, you must consider whether there is a threat to which type of design validity?

_____ 6. A year-long intervention study was conducted with first time mothers which compared the emotional responsiveness of their infants between the intervention group and the control group. Which type of design validity was threatened by the study methods?

_____ 7. Only 10% of the study participants withdrew from a study because of the time constraints and personal and family illnesses, which strengthens which type of design validity?

_____   8. Researchers and data collectors were blinded to the group receiving the diet educational intervention through a mobile application to strengthen this type of design validity.

_____   9. A diabetic educational program was developed with accuracy and consistently implemented with a protocol in a study, which strengthens what type of design validity?

_____   10. This type of design validity was strengthened by measuring pain using the Pain Perception Scale and the FACES rating scale.

Control and Designs for Nursing Studies

Directions: For each of the questions below, identify the **most** appropriate research design and provide a rationale for the design you selected. Each type of design or study is used only once. The designs are listed in order of control from the one with the most to the least control. After identifying the design, list one or more strengths of the study.

Designs from Which to Select
Randomized controlled trial (RCT)
Quasi-experimental pretest and post-test design with control group
Quasi-experimental post-test-only design with comparison group
Comparative descriptive design
Descriptive correlational study

1. A researchers examined the effect on acute pain of showing an animated cartoon on a laptop computer during the insertion of an IV in children 5 to 7 years of age. The sample was children undergoing scheduled surgical procedures such as tonsillectomy. The intervention group was recruited on Mondays and Wednesday and the comparison group was recruited on Tuesdays and Thursdays. Each group had 40 children (total sample 80). The children's acute pain scores were measured with the FACES pain rating scale immediately following the completion of the program and IV insertion.

   Design: _____

   Rationale: _____

   _____

   _____

   _____

   Study strengths: _____

   _____

   _____

   _____

2. A non-random sample of 100 first-time mothers was studied to examine the relationships among the variables of hours of sleep, stress level, anxiety level, and depression 1 month after the birth of their infants.

Design: _____

Rationale: _____

_____

_____

_____

Study strengths: _____

_____

_____

_____

3. A study was conducted to examine the effect of vitamins on weight gain in a sample of infants diagnosed with failure to thrive at 2 months of age. The sample of 90 infants was obtained from five pediatric clinics; 45 infants were randomly assigned to the intervention group and 45 to the comparison group. The infants were weighed before and after the implementation of the vitamin intervention, which lasted for 6 months. The sample size was determined by power analysis The intervention was implemented using a structured protocol.

Design: _____

Rationale: _____

_____

_____

_____

Study strengths: _____

_____

_____

_____

4. The study included a convenience sample of 150 women with Stage 3 breast cancer who received 4 weeks of radiation treatments. The women were recruited from three oncology centers with different treatment philosophies. One center emphasized wellness as part the of the treatment; another one included structured exercise; the last one ensured treatment side effects were aggressively prevented as much as possible. The differences in the women's perceived self-esteem, depression, anxiety, fatigue, and self-care among the centers were compared at 3 months post radiation treatment. The measurements used in the study were instruments with documented reliability and validity in similar samples.

Design: _____

Rationale: _____

_____

_____

_____

Study strengths: _____

_____

_____

_____

5. A study was conducted to examine the effectiveness of a new drug to treat hypertension compared to amlodipine in adults. The study had a sample of convenience and included patients with hypertension in the primary care clinics of a large healthcare system in Texas. Potential participants were carefully screened to ensure amlodipine or the new drug were safe treatments for their hypertension. The 456 participants were randomly assigned to either the intervention group or comparison group. The drug intervention was highly controlled to ensure accurate delivery of the medication, and blood pressures (BPs) were precisely measured at the start of the study and 3 months later. Participants, researchers, healthcare providers, and data collectors did not know which participants received the study medication and which received amlodipine.

Design: _____

Rationale: _____

_____

_____

_____

Study strengths: _____

_____

_____

_____

EXERCISE 3: WEB-BASED INFORMATION AND RESOURCES

Directions: Answer the following questions with the appropriate website or relevant information.

1. Nurse researchers should follow what guideline for developing, conducting, and reporting a RCT?

   _____

   Identify the website for these guidelines: _____

2. On the website you found in Question 1, review the Extensions section and find the extension for Social and Psychological Interventions. In what year was the extension for social and psychological interventions approved? _____

3. Identify the website for the National Institutes of Health (NIH) Grants & Funding.

   _____

   How much does NIH invest each year in biomedical research? _____

4. Identify the website for the National Institutes of Health (NIH) Research & Training.

   _____

5. From the NIH Research & Training page, identify the Medical Research Initiatives page.

   _____

6. From the NIH Medical Research site you found in Question 5, click on the Recover program for understanding the long-term effects of COVID-19. You will receive a warning that you are leaving the NIH website. Continue to the Recover website.

   What type of study designs would be appropriate for studying the long-term effects of COVID-19? Explain why.

   _____

   _____

   _____

   _____

   _____

   _____

7. The study conducted by Steffen et al. (2021) was registered at ClinialTrials.gov. Refer to the article in Appendix A. Use the registration number from the article, the disease that the participants had, and the country to search. Identify the webpage where the study is shown on the registration site.

   _____

   What is the status of the study as shown on the website? _____

EXERCISE 4: CONDUCTING CRITICAL APPRAISALS TO BUILD AN EVIDENCE-BASED PRACTICE

Steffen et al. (2021) Critical Appraisal
Directions: Examine the design of the Steffen et al. (2021) study in Appendix A, and answer the following critical appraisal questions about the design.

1. Identify the specific label or name that Steffen et al.(2021) used to describe their study design.

   _____

   _____

2. Critically appraise the intervention in the study.

   a. What was the intervention? _____

   b. Who delivered the intervention? _____

   c. What were the criteria to be selected to deliver the intervention? _____

   _____

   d. Describe the training that the persons who delivered the intervention received.

   _____

   _____

   _____

   _____

   e. How was the training evaluated? _____

   _____

   _____

   _____

   f. How would you evaluate the intervention fidelity?

   _____

   _____

   _____

   _____

3. Did the design include a comparison or a control group? Provide a rationale for your answer.

_____

_____

_____

4. Identify four aspects of the study methods which strengthen the design validity of the Steffen et al. (2021) study. State the action taken and which type of design validity it strengthened.

a. _____

_____

b. _____

_____

c. _____

_____

d. _____

_____

6. Identify two aspects of the study methods which were threats to design validity in the Steffen et al. (2021) study. State the problem and which type of design validity was threatened.

a. _____

_____

b. _____

_____

Greene and Ramos (2021) Critical Appraisal
Directions: Examine the quantitative component of the Greene and Ramos (2021) mixed method study in Appendix C, and answer the following critical appraisal questions about the noninterventional design.

1. Identify the type of design implemented in the quantitative component of the Greene and Ramos (2021) study.

_____

2. Was the design clearly identified? (**Yes** or **No**) Provide a rationale for your answer.

_____

_____

_____

3. How were the quantitative data collected and from whom?

_____

_____

_____

_____

4. From the limited information in the article, identify two design validity strengths in the Greene and Ramos (2021) study.

a. _____

_____

_____

b. _____

_____

_____

5. From the limited information in the article, identify two design validity threats in the Greene and Ramos (2021) study.

a. _____

_____

_____

b. _____

_____

_____

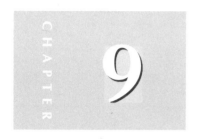

Examining Populations and Samples in Research

CHAPTER 9

INTRODUCTION

You need to read Chapter 9 and then complete the following exercises. These exercises will assist you in understanding and critically appraising the sampling process in published studies. The answers to these exercises are in the Answer Key at the back of the book.

EXERCISE 1: TERMS AND DEFINITIONS

Directions: Match each term below with its correct definition. Each term is used only once and all terms are defined.

Terms

a. Accessible population
b. Cluster sampling
c. Convenience sampling
d. Network sampling
e. Nonprobability sampling
f. Probability sampling
g. Purposeful or purposive sampling
h. Quota sampling

i. Simple random sampling
j. Sampling
k. Sampling or eligibility criteria
l. Stratified random sampling
m. Systematic sampling
n. Target population
o. Theoretical sampling

Definitions

_____ 1. Process of selecting a group of people, events, behaviors, or other elements that are representative of the population being studied.

_____ 2. Portion of the target population that the researcher can reasonably contact.

_____ 3. All elements (individuals, objects, events, or substances) that meet the sampling criteria for inclusion in a study.

_____ 4. Judgmental sampling that involves the conscious selection by the researcher of certain participants to include in a study.

_____ 5. List of the characteristics essential for membership in the target population.

_____ 6. Sampling method that involves selecting every *k*th individual from an ordered list of all members of a population, using a randomly selected starting point.

_____ 7. Category that includes all types of random sampling or when every member (element) of the population has a probability higher than zero of being selected for the sample.

_____ 8. Most basic probability sampling method that involves selection of participants from the sampling frame for a study.

_____ 9. Probability sampling method used when the researcher knows some of the variables in the population that are critical to achieving representativeness; the sample is divided into strata or groups using these identified variables and participants are obtained for each strata or group.

_____ 10. Probability sampling method in which the sampling frame includes a list of all states, cities, institutions, or organizations that could be in a study; a randomized sample of locations is drawn from this list and participants are obtained from the selected locations.

_____ 11. Snowball technique that takes advantage of social groups and the fact that friends tend to hold characteristics in common; participants meeting sample criteria are asked to assist in locating others with similar characteristics.

_____ 12. Convenience sampling method with an added strategy to ensure that a set number or percentage of study participants are included who are likely to be underrepresented in the convenience sample, such as women and minority groups.

_____ 13. Category that includes all types of nonrandom sampling methods or when not every element of the population has an opportunity for selection, such as convenience sampling.

_____ 14. A sampling method often used in grounded theory research to develop a framework, model, or theory through the research process.

_____ 15. Sampling method that involves including participants in a study because they happened to be in the right place at the right time.

EXERCISE 2: LINKING IDEAS

Directions: Fill in the blanks with the appropriate word(s)/response(s).

1. The individual units of a population are called _____.

2. The sample is obtained from the accessible population and is generalized to the _____ _____ if possible.

3. Representativeness means that the _____, _____ _____ and _____ _____ are alike in as many ways as possible.

4. Identify three ways you might evaluate the representativeness of a sample in a published study.

   a. _____

   b. _____

   c. _____

5. Is random variation in a correlational study sample a strength or weakness? Provide a rationale for your answer.

   _____

   _____

   _____

   _____

   _____

6. A list of every member of a population is referred to as a(n) _____

   _____.

7. A sampling plan outlines the _____

   _____

8. In critically appraising the sampling plan in a quantitative study, what three questions might you address?

   a. _____

   b. _____

   c. _____

9. When the sampling criteria are narrowly defined or very specific, the researchers desire a sample that is

   _____.

10. When the sampling criteria are broadly defined to include a variety of participants as in random controlled trials (RCTs), the researchers desire a sample that is _____.

11. Study participants must be over the age of 18, able to read and write English, newly diagnosed with colon cancer, and have no other chronic illnesses. These are examples of _____

    _____.

12. The sample was 65% female and 40% African American, 30% Hispanic, and 30% Caucasian. These are examples of _____.

13. When seven participants were lost to a study sample of 65 due to complications ($n = 3$), hospitalizations ($n = 2$), and diagnosis of additional illnesses ($n = 2$), what is the attrition rate for this example study? Critically appraise this attrition rate. _____

    _____

    _____

    _____

14. Identify four types of probability or random sampling.

    a. _____

    b. _____

    c. _____

    d. _____

15. Identify three types of nonprobability or nonrandom sampling commonly used in qualitative research.

    a. _____

    b. _____

    c. _____

16. Have the majority of published nursing studies to date used (**probability [random]** or **nonprobability [nonrandom]**) sampling methods? *(Circle the correct answer.)*

17. The adequacy of the sample size in quantitative studies needs to be determined by using _____

    _____.

18. Power is the capacity to detect _____ or _____
    _____ that actually exist in the population.

19. The minimal acceptable level of power for a study is _____.

20. Effect size is a specific numerical value used to represent the extent to which the _____
    _____ is false.

21. Identify three factors to consider when critically appraising the adequacy of a study's sample size in quantitative studies.

    a. _____

    b. _____

    c. _____

22. Identify three factors to consider when critically appraising the adequacy of a study's sample size in qualitative studies.

    a. _____

    b. _____

    c. _____

23. The two types of sampling criteria often included in a study are _____ and
    _____ criteria.

24. Calculate the refusal rate for a study in which 250 potential study participants were approached and 208 accepted participation in the study. What number and percentage of the potential participants refused to take part in the study? _____

_____

25. Calculate the attrition rate for a study with a sample size of 150 and 20 participants withdrew from the study (10 due to increased morbidity, 5 due to time constraints, 3 with transportation problems, and 2 due to mortality). What was the attrition rate for this study? _____

_____

Sampling Methods for Quantitative and Qualitative Studies

Directions: Match the appropriate sampling method with the example from a study. Some answer choices are used more than once.

Sampling Method

a. Cluster sampling
b. Convenience sampling
c. Network sampling
d. Purposive sampling
e. Quota sampling

f. Simple random sampling
g. Stratified random sampling
h. Systematic sampling
i. Theoretical sampling

Examples

_____ 1. A sample of 98 diabetic patients was obtained from an outpatient clinic then randomly placed in the comparison and intervention groups.

_____ 2. A sample of 500 nurses was randomly selected from a list of all registered nurses in the state of Texas.

_____ 3. A sample of 10 participants with human immunodeficiency virus (HIV) was obtained by asking three individuals to identify friends with HIV who might participate in the study.

_____ 4. A sample of 1000 critical care nurses was obtained by asking 100 critical care nurse managers in 50 randomly selected, large hospitals to identify 10 staff nurses to complete a survey.

_____ 5. A sample of 18 adults, who had received the COVID-19 vaccine within two months of its emergency approval, participated in a focus group to discuss their perceptions.

_____ 6. A sample of 120 study participants was obtained by randomly selecting participants from five levels of income.

_____ 7. The researcher obtained a list of all certified nurse practitioners, picked a random starting point, and then selected every 25th individual to participate in the study.

_____ 8. A sample of 117 individuals with hypertension was recruited from a primary care clinic to participate in a study.

_____ 9. An equal number of patients with asthma, emphysema, and chronic bronchitis were recruited from the local Better Breathers Chapter and asked to participate in a study.

_____ 10. The sample included 18 patients with a diagnosis of Type 2 diabetes mellitus; 9 were examples of strong self-care and 9 were examples of poor self-care.

_____ 11. A sample of 2500 military personnel was randomly selected to participate in a study.

_____ 12. A sample of 18 homeless, drug-addicted individuals was obtained by asking seven participants to identify other homeless individuals who were drug addicted.

_____ 13. A sample of 17 home health patients was asked to participate in a study because they had what were determined to be stage IV pressure ulcers that were not healing.

_____ 14. A sample of 150 adolescents was obtained at three fast-food restaurants.

_____ 15. A sample of 110 surgery patients was randomly selected from a hospital list and randomly assigned to either the control group or the intervention group.

_____ 16. Starting from a random point, every 10th participant who entered the emergency department was selected for participation in the study until a sample of 100 was achieved.

_____ 17. A grounded theory study was conducted to develop a framework, model, or theory about family members' perceptions to having a loved one hospitalized with COVID-19.

_____ 18. A sample of 120 heart transplant patients was obtained by asking 15 critical care nurse managers in 15 randomly selected, large urban hospitals to identify eight patients to participate in a study.

_____ 19. A sample of 85 participants receiving mental health care in a university health center was asked to participate in a study.

_____ 20. A sample of 12 participants who had experienced sexual assault was selected for a study; six of them were considered to be coping well after the assault, and six were considered to be coping very poorly after the assault. Data saturation was achieved with these 12 participants.

Determining Sample Size for Quantitative and Qualitative Studies

Directions: Match the type of research, quantitative or qualitative, with the criteria for determining the appropriate sample size for a study.

Type of Research
a. Qualitative research
b. Quantitative research
c. Both qualitative and quantitative research

Criteria

_____ 1. Sample size is adequate when saturation of information is achieved in the study area.

_____ 2. The scope of the study influences the sample size; a broad scope requires more participants than does a study with a narrow scope.

_____ 3. Power analysis is used to determine an adequate sample size for a study.

_____ 4. The quality and the depth of information obtained from the study participants are used to determine the sample size.

_____ 5. As control in the study increases, the necessary sample size decreases.

_____ 6. The more sensitive the measurement methods used in a study, the fewer the participants who are needed.

_____ 7. The more variables or concepts examined in a study, the larger the sample size that is needed.

_____ 8. The sample size needs to be large enough to prevent a Type II error.

_____ 9. Purposive sampling is a common method used to obtain an adequate sample size.

_____ 10. Simple random sampling is the strongest method of decreasing the potential for bias.

EXERCISE 3: WEB-BASED INFORMATION AND RESOURCES

Directions: Provide answers to the questions in this section.

1. Identify a website that has a power analysis calculator. Review the website to improve your understanding of power and power analysis in research articles.

   _____

2. Identify a YouTube video on qualitative sampling. Provide the URL.

   _____

3. Was the information you identified for Question 2 consistent with the information in your textbook (Grove & Gray, 2023)? Give an example.

   _____

   _____

4. What is the website for GeoPoll blog and the entry authored by Roxana Elliott (June 18, 2020)? Its title is Probability and Non-Probability Sampling.

   _____

5. What two types of probability samples are compared in a figure in the blog entry?

   _____

6. Identify the website provided by World Health Organization (WHO) that provides quick links to COVID-19.

   _____

7. Identify the webpage for Healthy People 2030 Objectives and Data.

   _____

8. Identify the website for the National Center for Health Statistics.

   _____

9. Which government agency hosts the National Center for Health Statistics?

   _____

EXERCISE 4: CONDUCTING CRITICAL APPRAISALS TO BUILD AN EVIDENCE-BASED PRACTICE

Steffen et al. (2021) Study
Directions: Review the Steffen et al. (2021) study in Appendix A to answer the following questions.

1. Identify the study population for the Steffen et al. (2021) study.

   _____

2. List the sampling criteria for this study. _____

   _____

   _____

   _____

3. Were the sampling criteria clearly stated and appropriate for the study? _____

   _____

   _____

4. How were individuals recruited for this study?

   _____

   _____

   _____

5. Was probability or nonprobability sampling used in this study? _____

   _____

6. What specific type of sampling method was used in this study? Provide a rationale for your answer.

   _____

   _____

   _____

7. Identify five sociodemographic and health history characteristics of the Steffen et al. (2021) study sample.

   a. _____

   b. _____

   c. _____

   d. _____

   e. _____

8. Is the sample representative of the target population? (**Yes** or **No**) Provide a rationale for your answer.

_____

_____

_____

_____

_____

9. What was the sample size at the start of the study? How many participants completed the study? Refer to Figure 1 on page e205.

_____

10. Using data from Figure 1, calculate the sample attrition rate for the study and for each group. Round your answers to the closest whole percent.

_____

_____

_____

_____

_____

11. Was a rationale provided for the sample attrition? Was the discussion of attrition a strength or weakness? Provide a rationale for your answer.

_____

_____

_____

_____

_____

_____

12. Was the sample size adequate? Provide a rationale that includes power analysis if it was conducted to determine the necessary sample size.

_____

_____

_____

_____

_____

_____

13. Can the findings be generalized to the target population? (**Yes** or **No**) Provide a rationale for your answer.

_____

_____

_____

_____

_____

_____

_____

14. What was the setting for this study? Was the setting natural, partially controlled, or highly controlled?

_____

_____

15. Was the setting appropriate for this RCT? (**Yes** or **No**) Provide a rationale for your answer.

_____

_____

Colwill et al (2021) Study
Directions: Review the Colwill et al. (2021) study in Appendix B to answer the following questions.

1. Identify the study population. _____

2. List the inclusion and exclusion sampling criteria for this study. Were these criteria appropriate for this qualitative study?

_____

_____

_____

_____

3. How were the participants recruited for the Colwill et al. (2021) study?

    _____

    _____

    _____

4. Was probability or nonprobability sampling used in this study? _____

    _____

5. What specific type of sampling method was used in this study?

    _____

6. Identify the sample characteristics for this study.

    _____

    _____

    _____

7. Did these sample characteristics provide a clear picture of the study participants? (**Yes** or **No**) Provide a rationale for your answer.

    _____

    _____

    _____

8. What was the sample size? _____

9. Was the sample size adequate? (**Yes** or **No**) Provide a rationale for your answer.

    _____

    _____

    _____

    _____

10. What was the setting for this study? Was this setting appropriate? (**Yes** or **No**) Provide a rationale for your answer.

_____

_____

_____

_____

_____

Greene and Ramos (2021) Study
Directions: Review the Greene and Ramos (2021) study in Appendix C and answer the following questions.

1. Identify the population for the Greene and Ramos (2021) study.

_____

2. What were the sampling criteria for the quantitative part of this study?

_____

_____

_____

_____

_____

3. Identify the sample characteristics for the Greene and Ramos (2021) study. What demographic variables were described?

_____

_____

_____

_____

4. Did the researchers provide a clear description of the sample? (**Yes** or **No**) Provide a rationale for your answer.

_____

_____

_____

_____

5. Was probability or nonprobability sampling used in the quantitative part of this study? What specific sampling method was used to select study participants?

_____

_____

6. What was the sample size for the quantitative part of this mixed methods study? Was this sample size adequate? (**Yes** or **No**) Provide a rationale for your answer.

_____

_____

_____

_____

_____

7. What were the sampling criteria for the qualitative part of this study?

_____

_____

_____

8. Were the sampling criteria clearly identified for the qualitative part of this study? (**Yes** or **No**) Provide a rationale for your answer.

_____

_____

_____

9. Was probability or nonprobability sampling used in the qualitative part of this study? What specific sampling method was used to select study participants?

_____

_____

10. What was the sample size for the qualitative part of this mixed methods study? Was this sample size adequate? (**Yes** or **No**) Provide a rationale for your answer.

_____

_____

_____

_____

_____

11. What was the setting for the qualitative part of Greene and Ramos (2021) study? Was the setting natural, partially controlled, or highly controlled? Provide a rationale for your answer.

_____

_____

_____

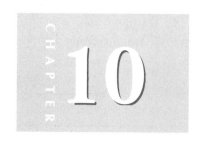

Clarifying Measurement and Data Collection in Quantitative Research

INTRODUCTION

You need to read Chapter 10 and then complete the following exercises. These exercises will assist you in learning key terms and identifying and critically appraising measurement and data collection procedures in published studies. The answers for these exercises are in the Answer Key at the back of the book.

EXERCISE 1: TERMS AND DEFINITIONS

Measurement Concepts and Methods

Directions: Match each term below with its correct definition. Each term is used only once and all terms are defined.

Terms

a. Direct measures
b. Indirect measures
c. Interval-level measurement
d. Interview
e. Likert scale
f. Measurement error
g. Nominal-level measurement
h. Ordinal-level measurement

i. Random measurement error
j. Rating scales
k. Ratio-level measurement
l. Structured observational measurement
m. Systematic measurement error
n. True measure or score
o. Visual analog scale

Definitions

_____ 1. Lowest level of measurement when data can be organized into categories that are exclusive and exhaustive, but the categories cannot be rank-ordered.

_____ 2. A scale that includes a 100-mm line with anchors on the extreme ends, which might indicate no pain before the left anchor and excruciating pain after the right anchor. Study participants are asked to mark through the line where they perceive their pain level to be.

_____ 3. Level of measurement with categories that can be rank-ordered, such as levels of self-care—below average self-care, average self-care, and above average self-care.

_____ 4. Ideal or perfect measure that does not include error.

_____ 5. Measurement method that requires observation of specific elements in a situation.

_____ 6. Scaling technique requiring patients to judge the level of their symptoms, such as a nurse asking patients to identify their level of pain on a scale of 1 to 10.

_____ 7. Error that occurs consistently in one direction, such as a scale that weighs everyone 2 pounds less than their true weight, that can alter study results, and must be minimized.

_____ 8. Level of measurement with equal numerical distances between the intervals and an absolute zero point.

_____ 9. Questions posed orally to a study participant as a way of collecting data.

_____ 10. Concrete variables (e.g., blood pressure (BP), oxygen saturation, and weight) involve these types of measures.

_____ 11. A multiple-item scale used to measure perceptions of a phenomenon in a study, such as a 20-item scale used to measure perception of depression with ratings of 1—strongly disagree, 2—disagree, 3—agree, and 4—strongly agree.

_____ 12. Level of measurement with equal intervals, but without an absolute zero.

_____ 13. Type of error that occurs when a scale has limited reliability and validity in measuring a concept such as self-care.

_____ 14. Measurement of abstract ideas (e.g., depression, dyspnea, and self-care) involves these types of measures, which are also referred to as indicators.

_____ 15. Type of error in which individuals' observed scores vary haphazardly around their true scores.

Reliability, Validity, Accuracy, and Precision in Measurement

Directions: Match each term below with its correct definition. Each term is used only once and all terms are defined.

Terms
a. Accuracy
b. Alternate forms reliability
c. Content validity
d. Evidence of validity from contrasting groups
e. Evidence of validity from convergence
f. Evidence of validity from divergence
g. Internal consistency reliability
h. Interrater reliability
i. Precision
j. Predictive reliability
k. Readability level
l. Reliability
m. Test–retest reliability
n. Validity

Definitions

_____ 1. Concerned with the consistency of a measurement method.

_____ 2. Addresses the extent to which the physiological instrument or equipment measures what it is supposed to and is comparable to validity for scales.

_____ 3. Determination of how well an instrument or scale reflects the abstract concept being examined.

_____ 4. Type of validity where two scales measuring the sample concept like depression are administered to a group at the same time and the study participants' scores on the scales should be positively correlated.

_____ 5. Repeated measurements with a scale or instrument to determine the consistency or stability of the instrument in measuring a concept.

_____ 6. Reliability testing used primarily with multi-item scales where each item on the scale is correlated with all of the other items to determine the consistency of the scale in measuring a concept.

_____ 7. Type of validity where an instrument or scale is given to two groups that are expected to have opposite scores, where one group scores high on the scale and the other scores low.

_____ 8. Comparison of two observers or judges in a study to determine their equivalence in making observations or judging events.

_____ 9. Examines the extent to which a measurement method includes all of the major elements relevant to the concept being measured; review of scales by experts adds to this type of validity.

_____ 10. Degree of consistency or reproducibility of the measurements made with physiological instruments or equipment; comparable to reliability for scales.

_____ 11. Type of validity where two scales that measure opposite concepts, such as hope and hopelessness, administered to study participants at the same time should result in negatively correlated scores on the scales.

_____ 12. Conducted to determine the study participants' ability to read and comprehend the items on an instrument.

_____ 13. Type of reliability involving correlation between different forms of the same instrument to determine their equivalence in measuring a concept.

_____ 14. The extent to which an individual's score on a scale or instrument can be used to predict future performance or behavior on a criterion.

Data Collection

Directions: Match each term below with its correct definition. Each term is used only once and all terms are defined.

Terms
a. Administrative data
b. Data collection
c. Data collection plan
d. Primary data
e. Secondary data

Definitions

_____ 1. Detailed plan of how the study will be implemented that is specific to the study being conducted and requires consideration of the common elements of the research process.

_____ 2. The actual process of selecting study participants and gathering data from them during a study.

_____ 3. Data that are collected for an initial or original study.

_____ 4. Data collected for reasons other than research, such as the data collected within clinical agencies.

_____ 5. Data collected during previous research, stored in a database, and later used in other studies to address research questions.

EXERCISE 2: LINKING IDEAS

Directions: Fill in the blanks in this section with the appropriate word(s)/response(s).

1. A fasting blood sugar is an example of what level of measurement? _____

2. A reliability value of at least _____ is usually considered a strong coefficient for a scale that has documented reliability and has been used in previous studies.

3. A patient has stage 4 breast cancer. What is the level of measurement for this demographic variable?

   _____

4. Ordinal data have _____ intervals, whereas interval data have _____ intervals.

5. A questionnaire is defined as _____

   _____

   _____.

6. The common analysis conducted to determine homogeneity reliability of a scale that has measurement at least at the interval level is the _____.

7. A newly developed multi-item Likert scale to measure hope was administered to a group of patients with depression and had a Cronbach alpha of 0.70. Was the scale (**reliable** or **unreliable**) in this example? *(Circle the correct answer.)* Provide a rationale for your answer: _____

   _____

   _____

8. When critically appraising the measurement section of a study, it is most important for you to examine the _____ and _____ of a scale.

9. If a study's measurement is not reliable, (**it is** or **it is not**) valid. *(Circle the correct answer.)*

10. Temperature is an example of _____ level of measurement.

11. A(n) _____ interview includes broad questions and is commonly used in qualitative research.

12. A(n) _____ interview is designed with specific questions to be asked by the researcher and is similar to a questionnaire, which are commonly used in quantitative studies.

13. Which has a higher response rate: (**mailed questionnaire** or **personal interview**)? *(Circle the correct answer.)* Provide a rationale for your answer.

   _____

   _____

14. Criterion-related validity is strengthened when a study participant's score on an instrument can be used to infer his or her performance on another variable or criterion. Identify the two types of criteria-related validity included in this text: _____ and _____.

15. Describe four situations that might result in error in researchers' measurement of study variables.

a. _____

b. _____

c. _____

d. _____

Measurement Error

Directions: Match the type of measurement error, which is most likely to occur in the following measurement situations. You will use the types of error more than once.

Type of Error
a. Random error
b. Systematic error

Measurement Methods

_____ 1. Blood pressure (BP) taken with equipment that consistently measures participants' BP three points high than the actual value.

_____ 2. Scores on drug calculation tests taken in the morning in a classroom.

_____ 3. Beck Depression Scale completed by patients prior to their annual physical.

_____ 4. Pulse oximeter inaccurately measures oxygen saturation 5% lower that the participants' actual value.

_____ 5. Body weight measured at a clinic when patients are fasting.

Levels of Measurement

Directions: Match the level of measurement with the variables or measures listed below. You may use the categories more than once.

Levels of Measurement
a. Nominal
b. Ordinal
c. Interval
d. Ratio

Variables

_____ 1. Body temperature

_____ 2. Gender

_____ 3. Research course grade of 85%

_____ 4. Educational level

_____ 5. Diagnosis of type 2 diabetes

_____ 6. Severity of illness level

_____ 7. Score from visual analog scale

_____ 8. Hemoglobin A1c value

_____ 9. Depression score obtained using the Center for Epidemiologic Studies Depression Scale

_____ 10. Registered nurse licensure exam—passed

_____ 11. Length of hospital stay

_____ 12. Diagnosis of COVID-19

_____ 13. Pain score from Wong-Baker FACES Pain Rating Scale

_____ 14. Body mass index (BMI)

_____ 15. Marital status

_____ 16. Severity of COVID-19 in the intensive care unit

_____ 17. Systolic and diastolic blood pressure

_____ 18. Income measured as: <$60,000; $60,000–70,000; >$70,000

_____ 19. Ethnicity/race

_____ 20. Hospital versus rehabilitation care

Scales

Directions: Identify the type of scale being presented in the following examples.

Type of Scale
a. Likert scale
b. Rating scale
c. Visual analog scale

Examples

_____ 1. Self-care measured with the Self-Care of Coronary Heart Disease Inventory. Respond to each item on the 5-point scale from strongly disagree to strongly agree.

_____ 2. Mark your current level of pain on the line below.

No Pain |————————————————————————————————| Most Severe Pain Possible

_____ 3. On a scale of 1 to 10, how anxious are you feeling about your surgery?

Sensitivity and Specificity

Directions: Answer the questions in this section.
Complete the table below on sensitivity and specificity.

Diagnostic Test Results	Disease Present	Disease Absent or Not Present
Positive test	*a* (true positive)	
Negative test		

1. What is the formula for sensitivity?_____

2. What is the formula for specificity?_____

Sensitivity and Specificity of Colonoscopy Screening Tests

Diagnostic Test Results	Disease Present	Disease Absent or Not Present	Totals
Positive test	250	50	300
Negative test	40	750	790
Totals	290	800	1090

3. What is the number of false positives for the colonoscopy screening test in the previous table? _____

4. What is the percentage of false positives for the colonoscopy screening test using the data in the previous table?

   _____

5. What is the number of false negatives for the colonoscopy screening test?

   _____

6. What is the percentage of false negatives for the colonoscopy screening test?

   _____

7. What is the sensitivity of the colonoscopy screening test? _____

   _____

8. What is your interpretation of the sensitivity value? _____

_____

9. What is the specificity of the colonoscopy screening test? _____

_____

10. What is the positive likelihood ratio (LR) formula? _____

_____

11. What is the positive LR for the colonoscopy screening test? _____

_____   _____

12. What is your interpretation of the positive LR value? _____

_____

13. What is the negative LR formula? _____

14. What is the negative LR for the colonoscopy screening test?

_____

15. What is your interpretation of the negative LR value? _____

_____

EXERCISE 3: WEB-BASED INFORMATION AND RESOURCES

Directions: Complete the following questions.

1. Identify the Agency for Healthcare Research and Quality (AHRQ) website for the EvidenceNow program:

_____

2. What is the purpose of the EvidenceNow projects within AHRQ?

_____

_____

3. Identify the website for the AHRQ that presents the priority populations for research.

_____

4. List the priority populations identified by the AHRQ: _____

_____

_____

5. Search for a national website that discusses the Center for Epidemiologic Studies Depression Scale-Revised (CES-R). Identify this website:

_____

Review the materials that are available on the CES-R.

6. There is a CES-R scale to screen children for depression. Locate a website that describes this scale:

_____

7. Identify the website for the Wong-Baker FACES pain rating scale: _____

_____

8. Steffen et al. (2021) examine blood pressure (BP) as one of the outcomes in their study. Whelton and colleagues (2018) published the most current source for the management of high BP in adults. What is the reference for this source?

_____

_____

_____

_____

9. Identify the website for the Health Reform Monitoring Survey (HRMS) that provided the data for the Greene and Ramos (2021) study.

_____

10. What is the purpose of the HRMS? What is the funding for this survey?

_____

_____

_____

_____

EXERCISE 4: CONDUCTING CRITICAL APPRAISALS TO BUILD AN EVIDENCE-BASED PRACTICE

Directions: Review the quantitative research article by Steffen et al. (2021) in Appendix A and the mixed methods study by Greene and Ramos (2021) in Appendix C and answer the following critical appraisal questions in the spaces provided. The measurement methods in the Colwill et al. (2021) study are described and critically appraised in Chapter 3 focused on qualitative research.

Steffen et al. (2021) Study

1. Identify the measurement methods for the dependent or outcome variables in the Steffen et al. (2021) study in the following table. Also indicate whether these measurement methods are direct or indirect method of measuring each study variable.

Variable	Measurement Method	Direct or Indirect Measurement Method

2. Present the information regarding the measurement of HbA1c as reported by Steffen et al. (2021).

_____

_____

_____

_____

3. Critically appraise the quality (precision and accuracy) of the measurement of HbA1c.

_____

_____

_____

_____

_____

_____

_____

4. Present the information regarding the BP measurements as reported by Steffen et al. (2021).

_____

_____

_____

_____

5. Critically appraise the quality (precision and accuracy) of the BP measurements.

_____

_____

_____

_____

_____

_____

_____

_____

6. What two variables were measured to examine their influence on the study outcomes (HbA1c and BP) in the Steffen et al. (2021) study? Complete the following table for these variables.

Extraneous or Confounding Variable	Name of the Measurement Method	Type of Measurement Method

7. Describe why Steffen et al. (2021) measured the variables in Question 6.

_____

_____

_____

_____

8. Identify the reliability and validity information of the Beck Depression Inventory presented in this research report. Critically appraise this information.

_____

_____

_____

_____

_____

_____

9. Identify some of the key ideas from the data collection process for the Steffen et al. (2021) study.

_____

_____

_____

_____

_____

_____

_____

_____

10. Critically appraise the quality of the data collection process in the Steffen et al. (2021) study.

_____

_____

_____

_____

_____

_____

_____

_____

Greene and Ramos (2021) Study

Directions: This critical appraisal focuses on the quantitative part of the Greene and Ramos (2021) study (see Appendix C). The qualitative part of this study is critically appraised in Chapters 3 and 14.

1. Identify the measurement method included in the quantitative part of the Greene and Ramos (2021) study.

   _____

   _____

2. Was the HRMS a quality survey? Provide a rationale for your answer.

   _____

   _____

   _____

   _____

   _____

   _____

   _____

3. Before using existing research data for a secondary analysis in a study, what actions should the researchers take? _____

   _____

   _____

   _____

   _____

   _____

4. According to Greene and Ramos (2021), how was trust measured in this study? What type of scale was used?

   _____

   _____

   _____

5. Describe key ideas from the data collection process for the Greene and Ramos (2021) study.

   _____

   _____

   _____

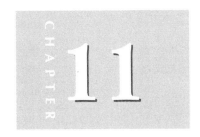

Understanding Statistics in Research

INTRODUCTION

You need to read Chapter 11 and then complete the following exercises. These exercises will assist you in learning key terms and identifying and critically appraising statistical techniques, results, and discussion sections in published studies. The answers to these exercises are in the Answer Key at the back of the book.

EXERCISE 1: TERMS AND DEFINITIONS

Directions: Match each term below with its correct definition. Each term is used only once and all terms are defined.

Terms

a. Alpha
b. Decision theory
c. Descriptive statistics
d. Effect size
e. Generalization
f. Implications for nursing
g. Independent groups
h. Inferential statistics
i. Outliers
j. Paired (dependent) groups
k. Post hoc analysis
l. Power
m. Probability theory
n. Type I error
o. Type II error

Definitions

_____ 1. Findings acquired from a specific study that are applied to a target population.

_____ 2. Summary statistics that allow researchers to organize data in ways that give meaning and facilitate insight.

_____ 3. Error that occurs with the acceptance of the null hypothesis when it is false.

_____ 4. Indicates the "degree to which a phenomenon is present in a population," such as the strength of a relationship between two variables, or "the degree to which the null hypothesis is false."

_____ 5. Level of significance that is set at the start of a study.

_____ 6. Theory used to explain the extent of a relationship, the likelihood an event will occur in a given situation, or the likelihood that an event can be accurately predicted.

_____ 7. Study participants with extreme values that seem unlike the rest of the sample.

_____ 8. Error that occurs with the rejection of the null hypothesis when it is true.

_____ 9. Theory with the assumption that all of the groups used to test a particular hypothesis are components of the same population relative to the variables under study.

_____ 10. The meaning of research findings for the body of nursing knowledge, theory, policy, and practice.

_____ 11. Groups are formed so the selection of one study participant is unrelated to the selection of other participants.

_____ 12. Data analysis after an analysis of variance (ANOVA) to determine differences among three or more groups.

_____ 13. The probability that a statistical test will detect a significant difference or relationship that exists.

_____ 14. Statistics designed to address objectives, questions, or hypotheses in studies to allow extension of findings from the study sample to the target population.

_____ 15. Study participants or observations selected for data collection are related in some way to the selection of other participants or observations.

EXERCISE 2: LINKING IDEAS

Directions: Fill in the blanks with the appropriate word(s)/response(s).

1. Identify the purpose of statistical analyses.

   _____

   _____.

2. List three steps that researchers conduct during the data analysis process to determine the results for their study.

   a. _____

   b. _____

   c. _____

3. List three statistical analysis techniques conducted to describe the sample characteristics in a study.

   a. _____

   b. _____

   c. _____

4. List five different types of results obtained from the statistical analyses conducted for quasi-experimental and experimental studies.

   a. _____

   b. _____

   c. _____

   d. _____

   e. _____

5. Identify five major ideas or content areas included in the discussion section of a research report.

   a. _____

   b. _____

   c. _____

   d. _____

   e. _____

6. Draw and label a normal curve with a mean of 0 and a standard deviation of 1.

7. In a normal distribution of scores, what percent of the scores fall between –1.96 and +1.96 standard deviations of the mean? _____.

8. The most precise level of statistical significance is achieved by conducting a (**one-tailed** or **two-tailed**) test of significance. *(Circle the correct answer.)*

9. A _____ error occurs if you say that a therapeutic touch intervention works to relieve acute pain when it does not.

10. An analysis of variance is conducted on study data to determine (**relationships** or **group differences**). *(Circle the correct answer.)*

11. The measure of central tendency calculated for nominal level data is _____.

12. A measure of dispersion that is calculated for interval and ratio level data is _____ _____.

13. What does "*n*" represent in a statistical table that includes the results from the intervention and comparison groups in a study? _____.

14. A diagram of points placed at the study participants' relative scores along a best fit line is called a(n) _____.

15. Data analysis that is conducted on two variables is called _____.

Linking Statistics With Analysis Techniques

Directions: Match each statistic with its appropriate analysis technique. Each statistic is used only once, and all analysis techniques have a statistic included.

Statistics

a. *df*

b. *SD*

c. α

d. *ES*

e. *R*

f. *F*

g. χ^2

h. %

i. *r*

j. *t*

Analysis Techniques

_____ 1. Alpha

_____ 2. Analysis of variance

_____ 3. Chi-square

_____ 4. Degrees of freedom

_____ 5. Effect size

_____ 6. Pearson product-moment correlation

_____ 7. Percentage

_____ 8. Regression analysis

_____ 9. Standard deviation

_____ 10. *t*-test

Linking Levels of Measurement With Analysis Techniques

Directions: Link the appropriate level of measurement for data to be analyzed by each of the following analysis techniques. The levels of measurement can be used more than once. Some of the statistical analyses can be used for two different levels of measurement. (Hint: Review Figure 11.8, Statistical Decision Tree or Algorithm for Identifying an Appropriate Analysis Technique, in your textbook *Understanding Nursing Research*, 8th ed.)

Levels of Measurement for Data

a. Nominal level

b. Ordinal level

c. Interval/ratio level

Statistical Analysis Techniques

_____ 1. *t*-test for independent groups

_____ 2. Chi-square

_____ 3. Mean

_____ 4. Pearson product-moment correlation

_____ 5. Percentages

_____ 6. Median

_____ 7. Regression analysis

_____ 8. Effect size

_____ 9. Standard deviation

_____ 10. Range

_____ 11. Mode

_____ 12. Ungrouped frequencies

_____ 13. Analysis of variance

_____ 14. *t*-test for paired or dependent groups

_____ 15. Grouped frequencies

Statements, Inferences, and Generalizations

Directions: Match the statement category with its example study. Each statement category is used only once.

Statement Categories

a. Decision theory statement
b. Probability theory statement

c. Inference
d. Generalization

Example Studies

_____ 1. The experimental pain assessment tool can be used to accurately assess pain levels in hospitalized adult patients after a variety of different types of surgery.

_____ 2. This type of statement suggests that when stress occurs, disruption in social activity and mood are likely to occur.

_____ 3. No significant differences were found in COVID-19 vaccination rates between two large cities in Texas.

_____ 4. Because most major risk factors thought to affect mental health did not change, and no adverse changes in sleepiness were observed during the intervention period, it is plausible to argue that the music intervention would not have reduced insomnia reports over longer time periods.

Describing the Sample

Directions: Referring to the table below, answer the questions that follow in the spaces provided.

Nurses (*N* = 100)	Frequency (*f*)	Percentage (%)
Age in Years		
18–29	10	10
30–39	20	20
40–49	35	35
50–59	30	30
60 and greater	5	5
Nursing Education		
Associate degree in Nursing (ADN)	40	40
Diploma	10	10
Bachelor of Science in Nursing (BSN)	50	50
Nurses' Years of Experience	Mean(*M*) = 15.5 (*SD* = 2.1)	Range = 1 to 35 years

1. Which variable contains grouped data? _____.

2. What is the mode of "Nursing Education"? _____.

3. Which "Age Group" is the median? _____.

4. What is the standard deviation for the "Nurses' Years of Experience"? _____.

5. What are the most years of experience that the nurses have in this example? _____.

6. Ninety-five percent (95%) of the nurses' years of experience are between what years? Round your answer to two decimal places.

   _____

   _____

Measures of Central Tendency

Directions: Referring to the results of a 10-item Likert scale with response options of 1 to 5, printed below, answer the questions in the spaces provided.

mean = 3.42   *SD* = 0.76
median = 3.10   mode = 3.00

1. Which value is the average? _____

2. Which value is the 50th percentile? _____

3. What does the mode represent? _____

4. Using the *SD* value, calculate the range of values ±1 *SD* from the mean. _____

   _____

   _____

Name That Statistical Analysis Technique!

Directions: Match the following statistical analysis results with the correct analysis technique. Identify the purpose of each analysis technique and the level of measurement (i.e., nominal, ordinal, interval, or ratio) required for conducting the technique.

Statistical Analysis Results

a. $\chi^2 = 4.61$ $df = 2$ $p = 0.10$
b. $t = 15.631$ $df = 180$ $p = 0.001$
c. $r = -0.315$ $df = 76$ $p < 0.05$
d. $F = 36.71$ $df = 420$ $p < 0.001$

Statistical Analysis Techniques

_____   1. ANOVA

       Purpose of analysis: _____

       Level of measurement of data analyzed with this technique: _____

_____   2. Chi-square

       Purpose of analysis: _____

       Level of measurement of data analyzed with this technique: _____

_____   3. Pearson product-moment correlation

       Purpose of analysis: _____

       Level of measurement of data analyzed with this technique: _____

_____   4. t-test

       Purpose of analysis: _____

       Level of measurement of data analyzed with this technique: _____

Significance of Results

Directions: In the following statistical findings, indicate whether the results were statistically significant (*) or not statistically significant (NS), assuming a level of significance set at alpha = 0.05. You may use each category more than once.
* = Statistically significant
NS = Not statistically significant

_____   1. $\chi^2 = 1.61$ $df = 2$ $p = 0.10$

_____   2. $t = 15.631$ $df = 180$ $p = 0.001$

_____   3. $r = -0.315$ $df = 76$ $p < 0.05$

_____   4. $F = 1.37$ $df = 25$ $p = 0.23$

_____   5. $R = .576$ $df = 130$ $p \leq 0.001$

EXERCISE 3: WEB-BASED INFORMATION AND RESOURCES

Directions: Answer the following questions with the appropriate website or relevant information.

1. Identify a website that provides a program for calculating power analysis for a study sample size or the power of a study results. _____

2. Identify a website for "Making Sense of Statistical Power" that will facilitate your understanding of power analysis.

   _____

3. What does SPSS stand for?

   _____

4. Identify a website that provides introductory information about SPSS:

   _____

   _____

5. The following workbook can provide you additional information about statistical analysis and assist you in critically appraising the results sections of published studies.

   Grove S. K., & Cipher, D. J. (2020). *Statistics for nursing research: A workbook for evidence-based practice* (3rd ed.). Elsevier.

   Locate this resource on https://www.amazon.com.

   _____

6. Find a website for Statistical Analysis System (SAS) for analyzing data.

   _____

7. Number Cruncher Statistical System (NCSS) provides statistical analyses tutorials, analysis software programs, and interpretation of statistical results. Locate the official website for this program.

   _____

EXERCISE 4: CONDUCTING CRITICAL APPRAISALS TO BUILD AN EVIDENCE-BASED PRACTICE

Steffen et al. (2021) Study
Directions: Read the Steffen et al. (2021) study found in Appendix A and then answer the following questions in the spaces provided.

1. How many groups did this study have, and what were the names of the groups? _____

   _____

2. How were the groups formed in the study? Identify the specific process.

_____

_____

_____

3. Were the groups independent or paired (dependent) in this study? Provide a rationale for your answer.

_____

_____

_____.

4. For each variable in the table, indicate the level of measurement (i.e., nominal, ordinal, interval, or ratio) and the descriptive analysis technique(s) that were conducted in the Steffen et al. (2021) study.

Demographic Variables	Level of Measurement	Descriptive Analysis Techniques
Sex (Gender)		
Age		
Race/Ethnicity		
Lives alone, yes		
Educational level		
Marital status		
Cardiovascular disease family history, yes		
Depression symptoms by the Beck Depression Inventory (BDI), positive score		
Smoking		
Consultation with a nurse in the previous year (yes or no)		

5. a. Were the Test/MI and usual-care groups significantly different for any of the demographic characteristics in the Steffen et al. (2021) study? (**Yes** or **No**) Discuss the results.

    _____

    _____

    _____

    _____

    b. If the two groups were not significantly different for selected demographic characteristics is this a study of strength or weakness? Provide a rationale for your answer.

    _____

    _____

    _____

    _____

    c. How did Steffen et al. (2021) manage any significant difference between the two groups for demographic characteristics?

    _____

    _____

6. In the following table, identify the level of measurement (i.e., nominal, ordinal, interval, or ratio) for each of the outcome or dependent variables and the descriptive analysis technique(s) that were conducted in the Steffen et al. (2021) study.

Outcome or Dependent Variables	Level of Measurement	Descriptive Analysis Techniques
Hemoglobin A1c (HbA1c)		
Systolic blood pressure (SBP)		
Diastolic blood pressure (DBP)		

7. What inferential statistic was conducted to analyze the differences between the Test/MI and usual-care groups for HbA1c, SBP, and DPB? (Hint: See the bottom of Table 2) Was this statistic appropriate? (**Yes** or **No**) Provide a rationale for your answer.

_____

_____

_____

8. What were the results for HbA1c between the Test/MI and the usual-care groups? What do these results mean?

_____

_____

_____

_____

9. What explanation or rationale did Steffen et al. (2021) provide for the HbA1c results in Question 8?

_____

_____

_____

_____

10. What were the results for SBP and DBP between the Test/MI and the usual-care groups? What do these results mean?

_____

_____

_____

_____

11. The following result was found on page e203 of the Steffen et al. (2021) study: "The test/motivational interviewing group showed significantly reduced HbA1c levels (0.4%) at the end of the study ($p < 0.01$)."

    a. Is this result statistically significant? (**Yes** or **No**) Provide a rationale for your answer:

    _____

    _____

    _____

b. Is this result clinically important? (**Yes** or **No**) Provide a rationale for your answer:

_____

_____

12. Were the results of this study similar to the results of other studies in this area?

_____

_____

_____

13. Briefly identify the limitations of this study? Do these limitations help explain the study findings?

_____

_____

_____

_____

14. Should these findings be implemented in practice now or is additional research recommended before use?

_____

_____

_____

15. What were the recommendations for further research? Do these seem appropriate?

_____

_____

_____

_____

Greene and Ramos (2021) Study

Directions: Read the Greene and Ramos (2021) study found in Appendix C and then answer the following questions in the spaces provided.

1. For each variable in the table, indicate the level of measurement (i.e., nominal, ordinal, interval, or ratio) and the descriptive analysis technique(s) that were conducted in the Greene and Ramos (2021) study.

Demographic Variables	Level of Measurement	Descriptive Analysis Techniques
Gender		
Age (ranges)		
Income (% of federal poverty level)		
Race/ethnicity		
Health insurance		

2. What was the design for the quantitative part of this study? _____

3. What type of inferential statistical analysis was conducted within the quantitative part of this study? What was the purpose of this analysis?

   _____

   _____

   _____

4. Trust in one's usual provider is correlated at 0.69 with the behavior "My doctor/provider listens carefully to what I have to say" for the full sample (Greene & Ramos, 2021, p. 1224).

   a. Is this correlation value significant? (**Yes** or **No**) Provide a rationale for your answer.

   _____

   _____

   b. Does the correlational value of 0.69 represent a weak, moderate, or strong relationship? _____

   _____

c. Is the 0.69 relationship positive or negative? What does that mean?

_____

_____

_____

d. What percentage of variance is explained by the 0.69 correlation?

_____

5. a. What was the lowest correlation value in this study? _____

   b. Describe this correlation identified in Part a of this question.

_____

6. Briefly identify the limitations in the Greene and Ramos (2021) study.

_____

_____

_____

_____

7. What were the main implication for practice? Were these appropriate?

_____

_____

_____

_____

_____

_____

8. What were some of the suggestions for further research?

_____

_____

_____

_____

_____

_____

9. Identify key conclusions from the Greene and Ramos (2021) study. Were these appropriate?

_____

_____

_____

_____

_____

_____

_____

_____

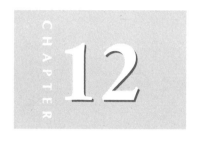

Critical Appraisal of Quantitative and Qualitative Research for Nursing Practice

INTRODUCTION

You need to read Chapter 12 and then complete the following exercises. These exercises will assist you in understanding the quantitative and qualitative research critical appraisal processes. The answers to these exercises are in the Answer Key at the back of the book.

EXERCISE 1: TERMS AND DEFINITIONS

Directions: Match each term below with its correct definition. Each term is used only once and all terms are defined.

Terms

a. Confirmability
b. Credibility
c. Critical appraisal
d. Dependability
e. Intellectual critical appraisal of a study
f. Qualitative research critical appraisal process
g. Quantitative research critical appraisal process
h. Refereed journals
i. Transferable
j. Trustworthiness

Definitions

_____ 1. Applicability of qualitative findings to other settings with similar participants.

_____ 2. Published collections of articles that have been critically appraised by expert peer reviewers.

_____ 3. Degree of readers' confidence that the findings from a qualitative research report represent the perspectives of the participants.

_____ 4. An appraisal process that includes identifying the steps of a quantitative study, determining the study strengths and weaknesses, and evaluating the credibility and meaning of study findings.

_____ 5. The extent to which a qualitative study is dependable, confirmable, credible, and transferable.

_____ 6. The documentation of the steps taken and the decisions made during data analysis in a qualitative study.

_____ 7. Examination of the quality of a study, event, or practice situation.

_____ 8. Extent to which other researchers can review the audit trail of a qualitative study and agree that the authors' conclusions are logical.

_____ 9. A rigorous, complete examination of a study to judge its strengths and weaknesses and determine the credibility, meaning, and relevance of the findings for nursing knowledge and practice.

_____ 10. An appraisal process that consists of (1) identifying the components of the qualitative research process in studies; (2) determining study strengths and weaknesses; and (3) evaluating the trustworthiness and meaning of study findings.

EXERCISE 2: LINKING IDEAS

Directions: Fill in the blanks with the appropriate words or responses.

1. Identify three important questions that are part of an intellectual research critical appraisal.

    a. _____

    b. _____

    c. _____

2. Identify at least three reasons why you would critically appraise nursing studies.

    a. _____

    b. _____

    c. _____

3. Adherence to ethical standards in nursing involves protecting study participants' _____ and obtaining _____ _____ from the participants.

4. In qualitative research, what components should be included in the abstract?

    a. _____

    b. _____

    c. _____

    d. _____

Determination of Quantitative Study Strengths and Weaknesses

Directions: Read the quantitative examples below and label each with **S** if it is a **strength** of the study or **W** if it is a **weakness** of the study.

Examples

_____ 1. The study framework lacks a link to the study variables' conceptual definitions.

_____ 2. The principal investigator conducted an online learning interventional study for participants who have diabetes mellitus, using funding from Sigma Theta Tau.

_____ 3. The hopelessness scale used in a study with multiple sclerosis patients was newly developed by the researchers for their study.

_____ 4. Researchers did not include a protocol for training the healthcare providers who implemented the study's counseling intervention.

_____ 5. The research design is linked to the sampling method, study instruments, data collection, and statistical analyses.

_____ 6. Network sampling was used to recruit study participants.

_____ 7. The findings from a replication study are consistent with the findings of previous studies but also added new information.

_____ 8. Power analysis conducted prior to data collection showed a need for 25 participants for each of the two groups. A total of 55 participants were recruited with 28 randomized into the intervention group and 27 into the control group.

_____ 9. Researchers reported three significant results without reporting the level of significance (alpha).

_____ 10. Stratified random sampling was used to recruit participants for an outcomes study.

_____ 11. A power analysis was conducted prior to the start of a randomized controlled trial (RCT). A total of 110 participants were needed for the study, previous research indicated a potential attrition of 20%, and 120 participants were recruited.

_____ 12. The study of handwashing cleansing agents in COVID-19 hospital units was a double blind RCT.

_____ 13. Of the 25 references cited in a quasi-experimental study focused on a weight loss programs, 5 (20%) were published within the 5 years of article acceptance and 7 (28%) were published within the 10 years of article acceptance.

_____ 14. Prior to data collection, the institutional review board (IRB) from the researcher's university granted approval for a study of directly observed therapy of tuberculosis in homeless individuals.

_____ 15. Nurses' incidences of medication errors were measured using a computerized medication delivery system and the patients' electronic health record.

Determination of Qualitative Study Strengths and Weaknesses

Directions: Read the qualitative examples below and label each with **S** if it is a **strength** of the study or **W** if it is a **weakness** of the study.

Examples

_____ 1. All of the references cited in the phenomenological research article were from peer-reviewed journals published in the last five years except for a book on phenomenology.

_____ 2. Researchers labeled the study as qualitative but did not identify the specific qualitative approach used.

_____ 3. The review of literature did not justify the study purpose because a gap in nursing knowledge was not identified.

_____ 4. Study interviews were audio recorded and typed word for word to create a verbatim narrative; then the transcript was checked by the researcher while listening to the recording.

_____ 5. The participant quotes included in the article of a grounded theory study did not clearly support the themes and the themes were inconsistent with the concept the researchers identified.

_____   6.   In a study of the lived experience of childhood abuse, the researcher described the study protocol if the adult participants became upset during the study interview, which included stopping the interview and calling a previously identified psychologist.

_____   7. ˙ Prior to data collection, for a study on the lived experience of frequent loss among pediatric hospice nurses, the researcher obtained informed consent and participants signed written consent forms.

_____   8.   The exploratory descriptive qualitative study was conducted by two experienced RNs with master's degrees in nursing, supported by a PhD researcher.

_____   9.   The 22 interviews lasted an average of 70 minutes, were audio recorded, and produced rich data that addressed the research problem.

_____   10.   The qualitative researchers indicated that they used a specific computer software during data analysis, but did not describe how inconsistencies or differences were resolved among the members of the research team.

_____   11.   The abstract of a grounded theory study included the study's purpose, grounded theory as the specific qualitative methodology, sample, and key results.

_____   12.   The researchers identified the inclusion criteria to be the ability to speak English and a diagnosis of hypertension and the exclusion criteria as being unable to speak English and not having a diagnosis of hypertension.

_____   13.   The study findings were linked to specific quotes or observations and the identity of the participants was protected by using pseudonyms.

_____   14.   Interviews with nurses participating in a phenomenology study about workplace culture were conducted in the breakroom on the hospital unit during the nurses' shifts.

_____   15.   The researchers realized after reviewing the transcript of the 18th interview that they had not found any new information and had reached data saturation.

EXERCISE 3: WEB-BASED INFORMATION AND RESOURCES

Directions: Search, locate, and review the websites identified in the following questions.

1.   The Quality and Safety Education for Nurses (QSEN) Project has defined quality and safety competencies for nursing and proposed the knowledge, skills, and attitudes (KSAs) to be developed in nursing pre-licensure programs for each competency. These KSAs are for students in baccalaureate programs who are seeking to become registered nurses (RNs). Locate the QSEN website for the pre-licensure KSAs:

_____

2.   Which QSEN (2020) competency is the most closely linked to understanding the research process and critically appraising studies?

_____

3.   Which evidence-based practice (EBP) attitude competency is focused on critical appraisal of studies?

_____

4. Which EBP skill is focused on reading, understanding, and evaluating studies?

_____

5. On the website for the CONSORT 2010 guidelines, find the flow diagram that should be included in reports of randomized controlled trials (RCTs): _____

_____

6. Identify the website for the Critical Appraisal Skills Programme (CASP) that provides useful guidelines and checklists for appraising studies with a variety of designs:

_____

7. On the website for the CASP checklists, identify the web address of the PDF checklist for RCTs that was updated in 2020?

_____

8. On the CASP website, find the checklist for critically appraising qualitative studies. What are the three questions that guide the appraisal?

_____

_____

_____

EXERCISE 4: CONDUCTING CRITICAL APPRAISALS TO BUILD AN EVIDENCE-BASED PRACTICE

Notes for Critical appraisal of Steffen et al. (2021) Study

Directions: Read the research article in Appendix A and conduct a critical appraisal of the Steffen et al. (2021) study. Review the answers to the critical appraisal exercises for Chapters 2, 4, 5, 6, 7, 8, 9, 10, and 11 related to this study. Makes notes regarding the strengths and weaknesses for the following steps of the quantitative research process. Use these notes to write a critical appraisal summary for the Steffen et al. (2021) study. Ask your instructor to clarify any questions that you might have.

1. Writing quality: _____

_____

_____

_____

2. Title: _____

_____

_____

3. Abstract: _____

_____

_____

_____

4. Research problem: _____

_____

_____

_____

_____

_____

5. Purpose: _____

_____

_____

6. Literature review: _____

_____

_____

_____

_____

_____

7. Framework or theoretical perspective: _____

_____

_____

_____

_____

_____

_____

8. Research objectives, questions, or hypotheses: _____

_____

_____

_____

_____

9. Variables: _____

_____

_____

_____

10. Research design: _____

_____

_____

_____

_____

_____

_____

11. Sample: _____

_____

_____

_____

_____

_____

12. Protection of human subjects: _____

_____

_____

13. Setting: _____

_____

_____

14. Intervention: _____

_____

_____

_____

_____

15. Measurement: _____

_____

_____

_____

_____

_____

16. Data collection: _____

_____

_____

_____

17. Data analyses: _____

_____

_____

_____

_____

_____

_____

_____

18. Interpretation of findings: _____

_____

_____

_____

_____

_____

_____

_____

_____

_____

19. Limitations: _____

_____

_____

_____

20. Conclusions: _____

_____

_____

_____

21. Nursing implications: _____

_____

_____

_____

_____

_____

22. Further research: _____

_____

_____

_____

_____

_____

_____

Critical Appraisal Summary for the Steffen et al. (2021) Study

_____

_____

_____

_____

_____

_____

_____

_____

_____

_____

_____

_____

_____

_____

_____

_____

_____

_____

_____

_____

_____

_____

_____

_____

Notes for Critical Appraisal of the Colwill et al. (2021) Study
Directions: Read the research article in Appendix B. Conduct a critical appraisal of the Colwill et al. (2021) study. Many parts of this study were critically appraised earlier in this study guide (see Chapter 3 focused on qualitative research).

1. Writing quality

_____

_____

2. Title

_____

_____

3. Abstract

_____

_____

4. Research problem

_____

_____

_____

_____

5. Purpose

_____

_____

6. Literature review

_____

_____

_____

_____

7. Study framework or philosophical orientation

_____

_____

_____

_____

8. Research objectives (aims) or questions

_____

_____

9. Sampling

_____

_____

10. Ethical considerations

_____

_____

11. Data collection

_____

_____

_____

_____

12. Data analysis

_____

_____

_____

_____

13. Results

_____

_____

_____

_____

_____

14. Interpretation of findings

_____

_____

_____

15. Limitations

_____

_____

_____

16. Conclusions

_____

_____

_____

_____

_____

17. Nursing implications

_____

_____

18. Future research

     _____

     _____

19. Quality of the study

     _____

     _____

     _____

     _____

     _____

     _____

     _____

Critical Appraisal Summary for the Colwill et al. (2021) Study.

_____

_____

_____

_____

_____

_____

_____

_____

_____

_____

_____

_____

_____

_____

_____

_____

_____

_____

_____

_____

_____

_____

_____

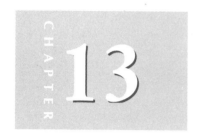

Building an Evidence-Based Nursing Practice

INTRODUCTION

You need to read Chapter 13 and then complete the following exercises. These exercises will assist you in reading and critically appraising research syntheses commonly published in nursing, including systematic reviews, meta-analyses, meta-syntheses, and mixed methods research syntheses. Exercises are also provided to assist you in implementing research evidence in your practice. The answers to these exercises are in the Answer Key at the back of the book.

EXERCISE 1: TERMS AND DEFINITIONS

Evidence-Based Practice Terms and Research Syntheses

Directions: Match each term with its correct definition. Each term is used only once and all terms are defined.

Terms

a. Algorithms
b. Best research evidence
c. Evidence-based practice (EBP)
d. Evidence-based practice centers (EPCs)
e. Evidence-based practice guidelines
f. Meta-analysis

g. Meta-synthesis
h. Mixed-methods research synthesis
i. PICOS question
j. Systematic review
k. Translational research

Definitions

_____ 1. A synthesis process of statistically pooling the results from previous quantitative studies using statistical analyses to determine the effect of an intervention or the strength of a relationship in a selected health-related area.

_____ 2. Clinical decision-making trees or figures nurses use when implementing research evidence in practice.

_____ 3. A structured, comprehensive synthesis of quantitative studies in a particular healthcare area or to address a practice problem to determine the best research evidence available for use in practice.

_____ 4. Highest quality research knowledge produced by the conduct and synthesis of numerous high-quality studies in a health-related area.

_____ 5. Patient care guidelines that are based on synthesized research findings from systematic reviews, meta-analyses, and extensive clinical trials; supported by consensus from recognized national experts; and affirmed by outcomes obtained by clinicians.

_____ 6. A format for initiating a research synthesis related to a clinical question that includes the following elements: population of interest, intervention needed for practice, comparison of interventions to determine best practice, outcomes needed for practice, and study designs.

_____ 7. Synthesis of the findings from independent studies conducted with a variety of methods (quantitative, qualitative, and mixed methods) to determine the current knowledge in a selected healthcare area.

_____ 8. Designated sites by the Agency for Healthcare Research and Quality (AHRQ) for the development of research in selected areas and the translation of the evidence-based findings into clinical practice.

_____ 9. A process and product of systematically reviewing, compiling, and integrating qualitative study findings to expand understanding and develop a unique interpretation of the studies' findings in a selected health area.

_____ 10. Type of research defined by the National Institutes of Health (NIH) as a methodology for promoting the use of basic scientific discoveries into practical applications.

_____ 11. Conscientious integration of best research evidence with nurses' clinical expertise and patients' circumstances and values in the delivery of quality, safe, cost-effective health care.

Evidence-Based Practice Models

Directions: Match each model with its correct definition and example. The terms can be used more than once.

Terms
a. Grove Model for Implementing Evidence-Based Guidelines in Practice
b. Iowa Model of Evidence-Based Practice
c. Stetler Model of Research Utilization to Facilitate Evidence-Based Practice

Definitions

_____ 1. A model developed in 1994 and revised in 2017 by a nursing collaborative that provides direction for the development of EBP in a clinical agency.

_____ 2. Framework developed by one of the authors of your text to promote the use of evidence-based guidelines in practice.

_____ 3. This is a comprehensive framework to enhance the use of research evidence by nurses in their practice that includes the phases of preparation, validation, comparative evaluation/decision making, translation/application, and evaluation.

_____ 4. The trigger might be an increased infection rate in a hospital and nurses might use this model to address this problem.

_____ 5. A new hand hygiene method is identified for implementation in an intensive care unit where care is provided to patients with COVID-19. Nurses using this model have the following decision options: not use (stop), use now, or consider using later.

_____ 6. This model was developed for using nationally recognized EBP guidelines in practice.

EXERCISE 2: LINKING IDEAS

Directions: Fill in the blanks with the appropriate word(s)/response(s).

1. List four benefits of developing an EBP for nursing.

    a. _____

    b. _____

    c. _____

    d. _____

2. Identify three sources you might access to keep current with the research literature.

    a. _____

    b. _____

    c. _____

3. Identify two challenges to accomplishing EBP in nursing:

    a. _____

    b. _____

4. Identify two reasons why nursing lacks the research evidence needed for implementing an EBP:

    a. _____

    b. _____

5. The Iowa Model identifies methods to integrate and sustain a change in practice. Identify two of these methods:

    a. _____

    b. _____

6. Identify and describe three ways that research findings might be translated or applied into nursing practice that were discussed related to Stetler's Model of Research Utilization to Facilitate Evidence-Based Practice:

    a. _____

        Description: _____

    b. _____

        Description: _____

    c. _____

        Description: _____

7. The evaluation phase of the Stetler Model of Research Utilization to Facilitate Evidence-Based Practice includes formal and informal measurement of outcomes for the following groups:

   a. _____

   b. _____

   c. _____

8. The comparative evaluation phase of Stetler's Model includes four parts: substantiating evidence, fit of the setting, _____, and _____.

9. NIH developed funding awards for translational research to improve the _____

   _____

   _____.

10. In 1997, the AHRQ established 12 _____

    _____ to promote the conduct of research, development of evidence-based guidelines for practice, and the implementation of translational research.

Understanding Research Syntheses

Directions: Match the particular type of research synthesis with the appropriate strategies used to conduct these syntheses. Some of the answers include more than one type of research synthesis.

Types of Research Synthesis
a. Systematic review
b. Meta-analysis
c. Meta-synthesis
d. Mixed methods research synthesis

Synthesis Strategies

_____ 1. Review that includes syntheses of a variety of quantitative and qualitative study designs to determine the current knowledge about medication administration technologies and patient safety.

_____ 2. Grey literature should be included in which types of research syntheses?

_____ 3. The systematic compiling and integration of the results from qualitative studies to expand understanding and develop a unique interpretation of women's experiences related to losing a child.

_____ 4. A structured, comprehensive synthesis of the research literature to determine the best research evidence available to address the following healthcare question: What are the best interventions to promote weight loss in adolescents? This synthesis might include meta-analysis and other types of research synthesis.

_____ 5. The PICOS format (**P**opulation, **I**ntervention, **C**omparison, **O**utcomes, and **S**tudy designs) is used to generate a clinical question to direct these types of research synthesis.

_____ 6. Meta-summary is the summarizing of findings across qualitative reports to identify knowledge in a selected area, and this summary is part of this research synthesis.

_____ 7. One type of research synthesis might use only randomized controlled trials (RCTs) and meta-analyses as sources.

_____ 8. Research synthesis that involves the statistical pooling of the results from previous studies into a single quantitative analysis that provides one of the highest levels of evidence about the effectiveness of music in promoting rest in an intensive care unit (ICU).

_____ 9. Ancestry searches use citations in relevant studies to identify additional studies. Which of these research syntheses use ancestry searches?

_____ 10. The reports from this type of qualitative synthesis might be presented in different formats based on the knowledge developed and the perspective of the authors.

_____ 11. Multilevel synthesis and parallel synthesis are two different approaches that might be used in conducting this type of research synthesis.

_____ 12. A funnel plot might be developed to assess for biases in a group of studies when conducting this type of research synthesis.

_____ 13. The synthesis of qualitative studies to describe the experience of postpartum depression.

_____ 14. Publication and reporting biases can weaken the validity of what types of research synthesis?

_____ 15. A preferred reporting statement called PRISMA has been developed to promote consistency and quality in the development of these two types of research syntheses.

Application of the Phases of Stetler's Model

Directions: Match the phase in Stetler's Model with the appropriate description and/or example. Each phase is used only once and all phases are identified.

Phases
a. Preparation
b. Validation
c. Comparative evaluation/decision making
d. Translation/application
e. Evaluation

Descriptions

_____ 1. The phase in which nurses evaluate the feasibility of using the Braden Scale to prevent pressure ulcers in their clinical agency.

_____ 2. The phase in which nurses develop a formal protocol for treatment of stage IV pressure ulcers in older adults.

_____ 3. The first awareness of the existence of an exercise program for severely disabled children obtained from attending a research conference and reading the study and similar studies in research journals.

_____ 4. Research knowledge about prevention of hospitalized infections is synthesized and evaluated using specific criteria.

_____ 5. The incidence of hospital-acquired infections is examined following the implementation of a new protocol to prevent infections.

Application of the Iowa Model of Evidence-Based Practice

Directions: Match the steps in the Iowa Model with the appropriate description and/or example. Each step is used only once and all steps are included.

Steps
a. Trigger issues or opportunities
b. State a question or purpose
c. Assemble, appraise, and synthesize body of evidence
d. Design and pilot practice change
e. Integrate and sustain practice change
f. Disseminate results

Descriptions

_____   1. The nurses were provided support to continue the fall prevention program and the number and types of falls were monitored through the hospital quality improvement program.

_____   2. A systematic review was conducted with 15 RCTs and a meta-analysis to identify an effective fall prevention program for the medical unit.

_____   3. Nurses and their manager noted an increased fall rate on their medical unit for the last two months.

_____   4. The results of the fall prevention program were communicated to the unit nurses and hospital administration.

_____   5. The nurses piloted the fall prevention program on just their medical unit.

_____   6. What interventions are currently used to prevent patient falls in the hospital? Are there more effective evidence-based interventions to implement to decrease the patient fall rate?

Agency's Readiness for Evidence-Based Practice

Directions: Think about the clinical agency in which you are currently doing your clinical hours. Provide responses to the following questions and discuss them in class or through your online discussion board.

1. Are the agency's policies, protocols, algorithms, and guidelines based on research? (**Yes** or **No**) Provide a rationale for your answer.

   _____

   _____

   _____

2. If you answered "no" to the previous question, what is the basis of the policies, protocols, algorithms, or guidelines of your agency?

   _____

   _____

   _____

3. Who are the individuals identified for promoting EBP changes in this agency? (Record the job titles of those involved.)

_____

_____

_____

4. Does the agency provide access to research publications for nurses? If so, provide some examples of these publications.

_____

_____

_____

_____

5. Does the agency have the goal of EBP? (**Yes** or **No**) If the answer is yes, what is the goal? _____

_____

6. Is the agency seeking Magnet status? What is the link of EBP to Magnet status?

_____

_____

_____

_____

7. Locate the following study:
Friesen, M. A., Brady, J. M., Milligan, R., & Christensen, P. (2017). Findings from a pilot study: Bringing evidence-based practice to the bedside. *Worldviews on Evidence-Based Nursing, 14*(1), 22–34. https://doi.org/10.1111/wvn.12195
This study might provide nurses guidance in promoting EBP in their clinical agency. What was the purpose of this study?

_____

_____

_____

_____

EXERCISE 3: WEB-BASED INFORMATION AND RESOURCES

Directions: Fill in the blanks below with the appropriate responses.

1. What does QSEN represent? _____

2. What is the website for QSEN competencies for pre-licensure or undergraduate nursing students?

   _____

3. List three EBP competencies in the *Skills* area identified by QSEN for undergraduate students.

   _____

   _____

   _____

4. The Oncology Nursing Society website (http://ons.org) has an "Explore Resource" section that includes putting research evidence into practice (PEP) information. Identify the website for EBP guidelines used to manage anorexia in patients with cancer:

   _____

5. Identify the Cochrane Library website that provides access to systematic reviews, meta-analyses, and integrative reviews of research.

   _____

6. Cochrane Nursing Care Field (CNCF) is part of the Cochrane Collaboration and can be found at http://cncf.cochrane.org/. Using that website, identify the site for the Cochrane Resources in Nursing:

   _____

7. Does the Cochrane Resources in Nursing include podcasts? (**Yes** or **No**) If yes, what is the website for the podcasts?

   _____

8. Locate the Nursing Reference Center (NRC) website. Identify the location for the Patient Education Reference Center on this site:

   _____

9. Identify the website for the U.S. Preventive Services Task Force's Recommendations: Information for Health Professionals.

   _____

10. The National Institute for Health and Clinical Excellence (NICE) can be accessed at what website?

   _____

11. Which website provides you access to the Joanna Briggs Institute located in Australia?

_____

12. Briefly describe the resources provided by the Joanna Briggs Institute?

_____

_____

EXERCISE 4: CONDUCTING CRITICAL APPRAISALS TO BUILD AN EVIDENCE-BASED PRACTICE

Directions: Read and critically appraise the systematic review and meta-analysis conducted by Saragih et al. (2021) to determine the global prevalence of mental health problems among healthcare workers during the COVID-19 pandemic. The critical appraisal guidelines for systematic reviews and meta-analyses are presented in Table 13.2 in your textbook, _Understanding Nursing Research_, 8th edition. The complete citation for the research synthesis critically appraised are as follows:

Saragih, I. D., Tonapa, S. I., Saragih, I. S., Advani, S., Batubara, S. O., Suarilah, I., & Lin, C. (2021). Global prevalence of mental health problems among healthcare workers during the COVID-19 pandemic: A systematic review and meta-analysis. _International Journal of Nursing, 121_, Article 104002. https://doi.org/10.1016/j.ijnurstu.2021.104002

You can locate this synthesis in the Research Article Library on the Evolve website for _Understanding Nursing Research_, 8th edition, at http://evolve.elsevier.com/grove/understanding/. Read this research synthesis and answer the following questions.

1. What was the problem statement for this research synthesis?

_____

_____

_____

2. What was the objective or aim of the systematic review and meta-analysis conducted by Saragih et al. (2021), and was it clearly presented?

_____

_____

_____

_____

_____

_____

3. What format was used for reporting this research synthesis? Is this a strength or weakness? Provide a rationale for your answer.

_____

_____

_____

_____

_____

_____

4. Was the PICOS format used to determine the inclusion criteria for this research synthesis? (**Yes** or **No**) If yes, describe the aspects of PICOS for this synthesis.

_____

_____

_____

_____

5. Was the search of the research literature rigorous and clearly described? (**Yes** or **No**) Provide a rationale to support your answer.

_____

_____

_____

_____

_____

6. Address the following questions regarding the research reports identified, screened, and included in the systematic review and meta-analysis.

    a. How many total citations were identified? _____

b. How many reports or studies were removed because they were duplicates? Discuss the significance of this.

_____

_____

_____

_____

_____

c. How many studies underwent full-text review? _____

d. What was the final number of studies selected for the systematic review and was the selection process detail? Provide a rationale for your answer.

_____

_____

_____

7. What was the focus of the meta-analyses conducted in the Saragih et al. (2021) research synthesis?

_____

_____

_____

_____

_____

8. Based on a meta-analysis what was the prevalence of post-traumatic stress disorder among the healthcare workers?

_____

9. How was the quality of the selected studies for the research synthesis assessed?

_____

_____

_____

_____

_____

_____

_____

_____

10. What were the main conclusions of this research synthesis regarding the global prevalence of mental health problems among healthcare workers during the COVID-19 pandemic?

_____

_____

_____

_____

_____

11. What were some of the implications for practice and recommendations for further research?

_____

_____

_____

_____

_____

_____

_____

Additional Evidence-Based Practice Projects

1. Conduct a project to promote EBP in a selected area of your practice. Use the following steps as a guide.

   a. Identify a clinical problem using the PICOS format that might be improved by using research knowledge in practice.

   b. Locate and review the research syntheses and studies in this problem area.

   c. Summarize what is known and not known regarding this problem.

   d. Select a model or theory to direct your use of research evidence in practice, such as the Iowa Model of Evidence-Based Practice or Stetler's Model of Research Utilization to Facilitate Evidence-Based Practice.

   e. Assess your agency's readiness to make the change.

   f. Provide education about the evidence-based change proposed to the nursing personnel, other health professionals, and administration.

   g. Implement the evidence-based change by a protocol, algorithm, or policy to be used in practice.

   h. Provide resources and emotional support to those persons involved in making the evidence-based change in practice.

   i. Develop evaluation strategies to determine the effects or outcomes of the evidence-based change on patient, provider, and agency.

   j. Evaluate over time to determine whether the evidence-based change should be continued. You might also extend the change to additional units or clinical agencies.

2. Use the Grove Model for Implementing Evidence-Based Guidelines to implement an evidence-based guideline from the Agency for Healthcare Research and other quality EBP websites into your practice.

   a. Identify a practice problem.

   b. Determine that there is an evidence-based guideline to address the practice problem.

   c. Examine the quality of the evidence-based guideline.

   d. Integrate the evidence-based guideline with nurses' clinical expertise.

   e. Use the evidence-based guideline in practice.

   f. Monitor outcomes (patients, families, health professionals, and healthcare agencies) from use of the evidence-based guideline in practice.

   g. Refine the evidence-based guideline as needed.

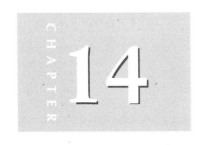

Introduction to Additional Research Methodologies in Nursing: Mixed Methods and Outcomes Research

INTRODUCTION TO MIXED METHODS RESEARCH

You need to read Chapter 14 and then complete the following exercises. These exercises will assist you in learning relevant terms and in reading and comprehending published mixed methods studies. The answers for these exercises are in the Answer Key at the back of the book.

EXERCISE 1: TERMS AND DEFINITIONS FOR MIXED METHODS RESEARCH

Directions: Match each term below with its correct definition. Each term is used only once and all terms are defined.

Terms

a. Convergent concurrent design
b. Explanatory sequential design
c. Exploratory sequential design
d. Mixed methods research
e. Pragmatism

Definitions

_____ 1. Study designs that use both quantitative and qualitative methods.

_____ 2. A study design in which quantitative and qualitative methods are both used and the findings of each set of methods are used to corroborate the findings of the other.

_____ 3. A study design in which qualitative methods are implemented first with the researchers using the qualitative results to design a quantitative phase of the study.

_____ 4. A philosophy that supports developing studies to solve problems by whatever methods fit the problem or question.

_____ 5. A study design in which a quantitative phase is followed by a qualitative phase and the qualitative results explain and expand the quantitative results.

EXERCISE 2: LINKING IDEAS FOR MIXED METHODS RESEARCH

Key Ideas for Mixed Methods Research

1. List two reasons why a mixed methods study may require more time to complete when compared to either a quantitative or qualitative study.

   a. _____

   _____

   _____

   b. _____

   _____

   _____

2. In the explanatory sequential mixed methods design, (**qualitative** or **quantitative**) data collection occurs first. *(Circle the correct answer.)*

3. What is another name for the convergent concurrent design?

   _____

4. Name five criteria by which mixed methods studies are critically appraised:

   a. _____

   _____

   b. _____

   _____

   c. _____

   _____

   d. _____

   _____

   e. _____

   _____

5. Draw a diagram representing the exploratory sequential design.

6. Describe how the diagram would be different for an explanatory sequential design.

_____

_____

_____

_____

Mixed Methods Research Methodologies

Directions: Match each methodology below with its correct description. Each methodology is used at least once and may be used more than once.

Methodologies
  a. Concurrent convergent design
  b. Explanatory sequential design
  c. Exploratory sequential design

Descriptions

_____ 1. The researchers asked participants to report their pain level each day for 10 days using a visual analog scale with a possible range of scores from 0–100. The data were analyzed and used to categorize participants as low pain, medium pain, and high pain. During the qualitative phase, participants in each category were interviewed and asked to describe their pain. Themes from each group were compared and descriptions of each type of pain experience were created.

_____ 2. While developing the proposal for a study, a team of researchers identified that quantitative researchers studying self-care efficacy had reported conflicting findings. To better understand the self-care efficacy of persons newly diagnosed with type 1 diabetes, the researchers administered a self-care efficacy instrument and asked participants whether they would be willing to participate in a focus group later. The focus group data collected a month later helped the researchers understand the research topic more fully.

_____ 3. The researchers conducted a series of three interviews with 22 persons newly diagnosed with renal insufficiency about the challenges to making lifestyle changes. Between the interviews, the participants were asked to complete a quantitative instrument about their perceptions of making lifestyle changes. The qualitative and quantitative data were analyzed separately and then combined to provide a comprehensive description of making lifestyle changes related to renal insufficiency.

_____ 4. A team of researchers evaluated instruments to measure symptom management of persons with multiple chronic illnesses. When they found none of the instruments were appropriate for their patients, they decided to conduct a mixed methods study. They conducted focus groups with their patients about symptom management. They analyzed the qualitative data and identified three themes. For each theme, they developed three to five items to measure symptom management using the focus group participants' words and phrases. The researchers then tested the instrument by administering the instrument to a national sample of persons with chronic illnesses.

_____ 5. A team of researchers recruited participants with early-stage heart failure for a mixed methods study and obtained informed consent. The participants were individually interviewed and then asked to complete a pencil-and-paper questionnaire on medication instructions and lifestyle changes before they left.

EXERCISE 3: WEB-BASED INFORMATION AND RESOURCES FOR MIXED METHODS RESEARCH

Directions: Search on the web for the following resources related to mixed methods research.

1. Find the document "Mixed Methods Research" on the website for the Office of Behavioral and Social Sciences Research, National Institute of Health. Provide the URL for the document:

_____

2. Who were the authors of the document found in Question 1? Provide their last names.

_____

_____

3. Find the document titled, "An introduction to mixed methods research" written by Tegan George in August 2021. Provide the URL.

_____

4. The document identified in the previous question is on a website sponsored by what company?

_____

When using web-based documents, you always want to determine the website sponsor. Notice that this type of website has advertising and may have biases in what is published. What the site provides may be accurate information, but the user must be aware.

5. John Hopkins University has been funded by the NIH to provide mixed method research training for health sciences researchers. What is the URL of the John Hopkins University Bloomberg School of Public Health that describes the training?

_____

EXERCISE 4: CONDUCTING CRITICAL APPRAISALS TO BUILD AN EVIDENCE-BASED PRACTICE

Mixed Methods Research

Directions: The study by Greene and Ramos (2021) will be used to answer the questions in this section. The article is available as Appendix C. Because several aspects of this study have been critically appraised in previous chapters of this study guide, these open-ended questions were selected from the Introduction, Integration, and Summary questions of the Critical Appraisal Guidelines for Mixed Methods Studies.

1. Was the research topic relevant and significant? Did Greene and Ramos (2021) explain what made the study relevant and significant?

2. What was the rationale for using a mixed methods design? Was the rationale adequately described?

3. Refer to Figure 14.1 in the textbook. Using the questions in the figure, what was the mixed method study design?

4. How were the results of the first phase used to refine the methods of the second phase?

5. Were the contributions to knowledge related to conducting a mixed methods study identified? If yes, what were the contributions? If no, what contributions can you identify?

_____

_____

_____

_____

_____

6. What were the weaknesses of the study? What were the strengths?

_____

_____

_____

_____

_____

7. Write a summary of the critical appraisal of the study. Include information from the questions you have just answered.

_____

_____

_____

_____

_____

_____

_____

_____

_____

INTRODUCTION TO OUTCOMES RESEARCH

You need to read the last part of Chapter 14 and then complete the following exercises. These exercises will assist you in learning relevant terms and in reading and comprehending published outcomes studies. The answers for these exercises are in the Answer Key at the back of the book.

EXERCISE 1: TERMS AND DEFINITIONS FOR OUTCOMES RESEARCH

Directions: Match each term below with its correct definition. Each term is used only once and all terms are defined.

Terms

a. Administrative databases
b. Clinical databases
c. Distal outcome
d. Nurses' roles in outcomes
e. Nursing Care Report Card
f. Nursing-sensitive patient outcomes

g. Outcomes research
h. Patient health outcomes
i. Proximal outcome
j. Quality of care
k. Standard of care
l. Structures of care

Definitions

_____ 1. These outcomes are influenced by nursing care decisions and actions.

_____ 2. These outcomes are clearly interwoven into the entire care context and include the following: symptom control, reduced complications, functional status, knowledge of disease and its treatment, satisfaction with care, and cost of care.

_____ 3. An established field of health research that focuses on the end results of patient care.

_____ 4. Databases that are created by insurance companies, government agencies, and others not directly involved in providing patient care.

_____ 5. Have three subcomponents that include nurses' independent role functions, nurses' dependent role functions, and nurses' interdependent role functions.

_____ 6. An outcome that is close to the delivery of care.

_____ 7. This includes a group of indicators that could facilitate the benchmarking or setting of a desired standard that would allow comparisons of hospitals in terms of their nursing care quality.

_____ 8. The elements of organization and administration, as well as provider and patient characteristics that guide the processes of care.

_____ 9. A norm on which quality of care is judged, such as clinical guidelines, critical paths, and care maps.

_____ 10. An outcome that is removed from the care or a service received and might be more influenced by external (nontreatment) factors.

_____ 11. The degree to which health services for individuals and populations increase the likelihood of desired health outcomes and are consistent with current professional knowledge.

_____ 12. Databases that are created by providers such as hospitals, clinics, and healthcare professionals.

EXERCISE 2: LINKING IDEAS FOR OUTCOMES RESEARCH

Key Ideas for Outcomes Research

Directions: Fill in the blanks in this section with the appropriate word(s)/response(s).

1. A theory that is commonly used as a framework for outcomes research was developed by

    _____ .

2. Identify the three aspects of person or patient health (see Figure 14.5 in your textbook, *Understanding Nursing Research*, 8th edition).

    a. _____

    b. _____

    c. _____

3. Donabedian identified three foci of evaluation in appraising quality of health. Identify these three foci and provide an example of each:

    a. _____

    b. _____

    c. _____

4. Nursing Role Effectiveness Model (see Figure 14.6 in your textbook) provided a framework for conceptualizing nursing roles. What do the nurses' independent role functions include?

    _____

    _____

    _____

5. Nurses' interdependent role functions include such actions as:

    _____

    _____

    _____

6. To evaluate an outcome as defined by Donabedian, the identified outcomes must be clearly linked to the _____ that caused the outcome.

7. List three examples of standards of care:

    a. _____

    b. _____

    c. _____

8. **Heterogeneous** or **Homogeneous** samples are preferred in outcomes studies. *(Circle the correct answer.)*

9. From an outcomes research perspective, identify three questions nurse researchers might address in conducting outcomes studies:

   a. _____

   b. _____

   c. _____

10. What are two types of databases that are important sources of data for outcomes research?

   a. _____

   b. _____

11. An extensive classification of nursing outcomes is being developed at the University of Iowa, College of Nursing. What is the name of this classification system?

   _____

12. Statistical methods for outcomes studies focus on analysis of _____
   and _____.

13. What are the three major questions used for critically appraising outcomes studies?

   a. _____

   b. _____

   c. _____

Outcomes Research Methodologies

Directions: Match each methodology below with its correct description. Each methodology is used only once and all methodologies are described.

Methodologies
a. Population-based studies
b. Prospective cohort study
c. Retrospective cohort study
d. Secondary data analysis
e. Standardized mortality ratio (SMR)

Descriptions

_____ 1. A study that involves any re-analysis of data collected by another researcher or organization, including analysis of data sets collected from a variety of sources.

_____ 2. An epidemiological study in which the researcher identifies a group of people who have experienced a particular event for investigation, such as an infection following a surgical procedure.

_____ 3. The observed number of deaths are divided by the expected number of deaths and multiplied by 100.

_____ 4. An epidemiological study where researchers identify a group of people who are at risk for experiencing a particular event and then follow them over time to observe whether the event occurs, such as the incidence of health problems in morbidly obese individuals.

_____ 5. Studies conducted within the context of the patients' community rather than the context of the medical system, such as the elderly individuals' physical and psychological functional levels in their homes.

EXERCISE 3: WEB-BASED INFORMATION AND RESOURCES FOR OUTCOMES RESEARCH

Directions: Identify the agencies, institutes, and databases that have contributed to the conducted of outcomes research. Provide the websites and other information to address the questions in this section.

1. AHRQ

    Full name: _____

    Website: _____

2. AHRQ supports the conduct and dissemination of outcomes research through what institute:

    _____

3. Identify a website for PCORI, an important outcomes research resource:

    _____

4. Identify the website for the vision and mission of PCORI? _____

    _____

5. What is the vision and mission for PCORI?

    _____

    _____

    _____

    _____

6. NQF

    Full name: _____

    Website: _____

7. Identify the website for the National Database of Nursing Quality Indicators (NDNQI) that is now managed by Press Ganey. (Hint: Search nursing quality)

    Website: _____

8. Which nursing organization established the NDNQI?

    _____

9. Identify a YouTube video about nurse sensitive outcomes or indicators.

    _____

10. Identify the website for Nursing Outcomes Classification (NOC) at the University of Iowa College of Nursing.

    _____

EXERCISE 4: CONDUCTING CRITICAL APPRAISALS TO BUILD AN EVIDENCE-BASED PRACTICE

Outcomes Research

Directions: The questions for this section address the Jeong et al. (2020) study that can be found in the Research Article Library for the Grove and Gray (2023) *Understanding Nursing Research* text. The complete citation for this study is provided as follows so you can also obtain it online. You need to read this article in detail and identify the steps of this outcomes study. Then answer the following questions.

Jeong, A., Lapenskie, J., Talarico, R., Hsu, A. T., & Tanuseputro, P. (2020). Health outcomes of immigrants in nursing homes: A population-based retrospective cohort study in Ontario, Canada. *JAMDA, 21*, 740-746. https://doi.org/10.1016/j.jamda.2020.03.00

1. Identify the problem and purpose for the Jeong et al. (2020) study.

    _____

    _____

    _____

    _____

2. What outcomes research methods were implemented by Jeong et al. (2020)?

    _____

    _____

3. Were the methods in this study clearly identified? (**Yes** or **No**) Provide a rationale for your answer.

    _____

    _____

    _____

    _____

4. Identify the outcome variables examined in this study:

_____

_____

_____

_____

5. Provide an operational definition for the outcome location of death.

_____

_____

6. Was a secondary data analysis conducted to address the study purpose? (**Yes** or **No**)

7. What were the sources for the data examined in this outcomes study?

_____

_____

_____

8. What was the sample size for this study? Critically appraise the sample of this study.

_____

_____

_____

_____

_____

9. What was the setting for this study? Critically appraise this study setting.

_____

_____

_____

10. What were the conclusions identified by Jeong et al. (2020) in their research report?

_____

_____

_____

_____

_____

11. What were the implications for practice and did they seem appropriate?

_____

_____

_____

_____

_____

12. Critically appraise the quality of this outcomes study.

_____

_____

_____

_____

_____

_____

_____

_____

_____

_____

Answer Key to Study Guide Exercises

CHAPTER 1—INTRODUCTION TO NURSING RESEARCH AND ITS IMPORTANCE IN BUILDING AN EVIDENCE-BASED PRACTICE

EXERCISE 1: TERMS AND DEFINITIONS

Acquiring Knowledge and Research Methods

1.	h	9.	p
2.	e	10.	b
3.	j	11.	i
4.	n	12.	k
5.	c	13.	d
6.	g	14.	o
7.	f	15.	a
8.	l	16.	m

Evidence-Based Practice Terms

1. d
2. e
3. a
4. c
5. b

Synthesizing Research Evidence

1. d
2. a
3. c
4. b

EXERCISE 2: LINKING IDEAS

How Research Influences Practice

1. Description involves identifying the nature and attributes of nursing phenomena. Descriptive knowledge generated through research can be used to identify and describe what exists in nursing practice, to discover new information, and to classify information of use in the discipline.

Examples: The answers can be any of the following or similar studies. a. Identifying the signs and symptoms for making the nursing diagnosis of acute pain. b. Describing women who are at risk for heart failure. c. Describing the incidence and spread of COVID-19 in 3 states.

2. Explanation focuses on identifying and clarifying the strength and nature of relationships among variables or concepts relevant for practice.
Example: Answers could be any of the following or other studies that involve relationships. a. Determining the relationships among medication adherence, social support, physical functioning, and energy among women post myocardial infarction. b. Examining the relationships between health promotion behaviors, such as diet, exercise, and sleep. c. Determining the association among perceived health equity and access to primary care.

3. Prediction involves estimating the probability of a specific outcome in a given situation.
Example: Answers could be any of the following or other studies that involve probability of an outcome. a. Likelihood of a septic patient having skin breakdown on an air-flotation mattress. b. Probability of new graduate nurses staying employed with the same hospital for at least five years. c. Probability of nursing students passing the NCLEX exam on the first attempt.

4. Control is the ability to manipulate a situation to produce the desired outcomes in practice. Therefore, nurses could prescribe certain interventions to help patients and families achieve quality outcomes.
Example: a. Implementing a protocol for the care of urinary catheters based on evidence-based guidelines to decrease the incidence of urinary tract infections. b. Determining the effectiveness of a clinical guideline for diabetic teaching in your institution. c. Based on the conclusions of systematic review, create a work environment conducive to nurses' mental health.

Historical Events Influencing Nursing Research

1. Florence Nightingale
2. *Nursing Research*
3. You might list any three of the following journals or identify other research journals published in nursing:
   Advances in Nursing Science
   Applied Nursing Research
   Biological Research for Nursing
   Clinical Nursing Research
   Journal of Nursing Scholarship
   Nursing Research
   Nursing Science Quarterly
   Qualitative Health Research
   Research in Nursing & Health
   Scholarly Inquiry for Nursing Practice
   Western Journal of Nursing Research
   Worldviews on Evidence-Based Nursing
4. Sigma or Sigma Theta Tau
5. 1985
6. National Institute of Nursing Research (NINR)
7. International North American Nursing Diagnosis Association (NANDA-I)
8. Agency for Healthcare Research and Quality (AHRQ)
9. *2030*
10. American Nurses Credentialing Center

Acquiring Knowledge in Nursing

1. You could have identified any of the following ways of acquiring knowledge in nursing. The following examples of each way of acquiring nursing knowledge are correct, but other examples may also be correct. If in doubt, compare your examples to those in the textbook.
   a. Tradition: nurses who are completing their shift giving report about their patients to nurses starting their shift; taking all patients' vital signs at 4 AM.
   b. Authority: ~~continue~~ implementing an intervention because expert clinical nurses, educators, or authors of articles or books indicate the intervention is the best.
   c. Borrowing: using knowledge from medicine, psychology, or sociology in nursing practice; assessing a family's dynamics using a theory from sociology; adopt a therapeutic communication strategy that was developed by psychologists.
   d. Trial and error: trying different medications to alleviate a patient's pain during burn debridement; positioning a patient confined to bed in different ways to reduce his or her discomfort; trying different interventions to help patients sleep in the Intensive Care Unit (ICU).
   e. Personal experience: learning by doing or experiencing; a nurse who has lost a family member understands how to comfort other families suffering loss; an Asian nurse who has experienced prejudice is sensitive to ways that other nurses are prejudiced toward patients of different races and ethnicities.
   f. Intuition: recognizing the moral distress of a new nurse; knowing that a patient's condition is deteriorating; recognizing that a patient's anxiety is about to escalate into panic. In each case, you have limited concrete data to support this feeling or hunch.
   g. Professional practice: developing strategies to relieve a patient's discomfort because you have done it before; knowing how to quickly arrange the supplies for a dressing change; starting an intravenous infusion in a patient with low blood pressure.
2. personal or professional experience
3. a. novice
   b. advanced beginner
   c. competent
   d. proficient
   e. expert
4. Research, empirical, or scientific
5. intuition
6. Deductive reasoning
7. You might identify any of the following outcomes that may be examined in outcomes research: patients' responses to intervention; health status (signs, symptoms, functional status, morbidity, mortality); patient satisfaction; costs related to health care; quality of care
8. Qualitative
   Gordon, J., Magbee, T., & Yoder, L. (2021). The experiences of critical care nurses caring for patients with COVID-19 during the 2020 pandemic: A qualitative study. *Applied Nursing Research, 59,* Article 151418. https://doi.org/10.1016/j.apnr.2021.151418
9. Outcomes research. You might have answered 'quantitative,' which is also true. However, the best answer is outcomes research.
10. Quantitative

Linking Research Methods to Types of Research

1. b
2. b
3. a
4. b
5. a
6. a
7. a
8. b

Nurses' Roles in Research

1. a. b.
2. a.
3. b. c.
4. e.
5. a, b, c, d, and e
6. d.

Determining the Strength of Levels of Research Evidence

Levels of research evidence are IV, I, V, II, VII, VI, and III.

EXERCISE 3: WEB-BASED INFORMATION AND RESOURCES

1. Dr. Loretta Sweet Jemmot; found at https://www.ninr.nih.gov/milestones-in-ninr-history
2. Equity; found at https://www.ahrq.gov/news/special-emphasis-notice.html
3. 4th edition; https://www.nationalcoalitionhpc.org/ncp/
4. https://health.gov/healthypeople/tools-action/browse-evidence-based-resources#social-determinants-of-health
5. Any of these answers are correct: Economic Stability, Health Care Access and Quality, Neighborhood and Built Environment, or Social and Community Context
6. "Integrate best current evidence with clinical expertise and patient/family preferences and values for delivery of optimal health care;" found at https://qsen.org/competencies/pre-licensure-ksas/#evidence-based_practice
7. The definitions are the same. The text indicates EBP involves the integration of best research evidence, clinical expertise, and patient's circumstances and values. In addition to the definition provided in the chapter, these components are identified in Fig. 1.1.

EXERCISE 4: CONDUCTING CRITICAL APPRAISALS TO BUILD AN EVIDENCE-BASED PRACTICE

Steffen et al. (2021)
1. Type 2 diabetes mellitus (T2DM) and arterial hypertension (AH)
2. ~~Chronic Care Model~~ June 2018-July 2019
3. ~~80~~ 3
4. ~~8~~ 94
5. ~~Deleted previous answer~~ Dr. Faustino-Silva

Colwill et al. (2021)
1. 5- all of them
2. Cleveland Clinic is a healthcare system with numerous locations including hospitals. Hospitals are considered inpatient settings, which was the term used by the researchers to describe the settings.
~~Deleted all answers for 3, 4, and 5 and replaced text with red font~~
3. grounded theory
4. endocarditis
5. *Applied Nursing Research*

Greene & Ramos (2021)
1. Health Reform Monitoring Survey or nationally representative survey
2. Telephone interviews; 40
3. ~~Deleted previous number~~ 6517
4. ~~Deleted previous answer~~ New York
5. 8 survey items

CHAPTER 2—INTRODUCTION TO QUANTITATIVE RESEARCH

EXERCISE 1: TERMS AND DEFINITIONS

1. l
2. s
3. a
4. d
5. r
6. n
7. h
8. k
9. q
10. j
11. m
12. c
13. f
14. t
15. b
16. g
17. e
18. p
19. i
20. o

EXERCISE 2: LINKING IDEAS

Control in Quantitative Research

1. highly controlled or laboratory
2. descriptive and correlational
3. quasi-experimental and experimental
4. random
5. nonrandom or nonprobability; random or probability
6. natural
7. natural or partially controlled
8. experimental
9. partially controlled
10. quasi-experimental and experimental

Steps of the Research Process

1. problem-solving process; nursing
2. Step 1: Research problem and purpose

Step 2: Literature review

Step 3: Research framework

Step 4: Research objectives, questions, or hypotheses

Step 5: Study variables

Step 6: Research design

Step 7: Population and sample

Step 8: Methods of measurement

Step 9: Data collection

Step 10: Data analysis and results

Step 11: Interpretation of research outcomes: Determining study findings, identifying study limitations, exploring the significance of the findings, forming conclusions, generalizing the findings, considering the implications for nursing, and suggesting further studies.

3. You could identify any of the following assumptions or other assumptions you have noted in research reports.

   a. People want to assume control of their own health and manage their health problems.

   b. Stress should be avoided.

   c. Health is a priority for most people.

   d. People who live in poor areas feel underserved for health care.

   e. Attitudes can be measured with a scale.

   f. Most measurable attitudes are held strongly enough to direct behavior.

   g. Health professionals view health care in a manner different from laypersons.

   h. Human biological and chemical factors show less variation than do cultural and social factors.

   i. People operate on the basis of cognitive information.

   j. Increased knowledge about an event lowers anxiety about the event.

   k. Receipt of health care at home is preferable to receipt of care in an institution.

4. You could identify any of the following reasons for conducting a pilot study:

   a. To determine whether the proposed study is feasible (e.g., Are the study participants available? Does the researcher have the time and money to conduct the study?)

   b. To develop or refine a research treatment or intervention

   c. To develop a protocol for the implementation of an intervention

   d. To identify problems with the design

   e. To determine whether the sample is representative of the population or whether the sampling technique is effective

   f. To examine the reliability and validity of the measurement methods to be used in a study

   g. To examine the precision and accuracy of physiological measures

   h. To develop or refine data collection instruments

   i. To refine the data collection and analysis plan

   j. To give the researcher experience with the study participants, setting, methodology, and methods of measurement

   k. To try out data analysis techniques

5. limitations

   (Koyuncu, A., Yava, A., Yamak, B., & Orhan, N. (2021). Effect of family presence on stress response after bypass surgery. *Heart & Lung*, *50*(2), 193-201. https://doi.org/10.1016/j.hrtlng.2020.11.006)

Reading Research Reports

1. You could identify any of the following nursing research journals.

   a. *Advances in Nursing Science*

   b. *Applied Nursing Research*

   c. *Biological Research for Nursing*

   d. *Clinical Nursing Research*

   e. *Journal of Nursing Measurement*

   f. *Journal of Nursing Scholarship*

   g. *International Journal of Nursing Studies*

   h. *International Journal of Nursing Terminologies and Classifications*

   i. *Nursing Research*

   j. *Nursing Science Quarterly*

   k. *Qualitative Nursing Research*

   l. *Research in Nursing & Health*

   m. *Scholarly Inquiry for Nursing Practice*

   n. *Western Journal of Nursing Research*

   o. *Worldviews on Evidence-Based Nursing*

2. Look in clinical journals and see which ones have several research articles in each issue. You might have identified any of the following or other nursing clinical journals:

   a. *Geriatric Nursing*

   b. *Oncology Nursing Forum*

   c. *Nephrology Nursing*

   d. *Issues in Comprehensive Pediatric Nursing*

   e. *Journal of Transcultural Nursing*

   f. *Heart & Lung*

   g. *Journal of Nursing Education*

   h. *Birth*

   i. *Nursing Diagnosis*

   j. *Public Health Nursing*

   k. *The Diabetes Educator*

   l. *Maternal-Child Nursing Journal*

   m. *Journal of Nursing Education*

   n. *Journal of Pediatric Nursing*

   o. *Archives of Psychiatric Nursing*

3. Major sections of a research report
   a. Introduction
   b. Methods
   c. Results
   d. Discussion
4. You might have identified any of the following that are included in the Methods section of a research report.
   a. Design
   b. Sample
   c. Setting
   d. Informed consent process
   e. Review of the study by institutional review boards
   f. Methods of measurement
   g. Data collection process
   h. Usually identifies the data analysis techniques to be conducted
   i. The methods section also includes the intervention if that is applicable to the type of study being conducted, such as for quasi-experimental and experimental studies.
5. You might have identified any of the following elements of the Discussion section of a research report.
   a. Major findings
   b. Link of findings to previous study findings
   c. Limitations of the study
   d. Conclusions drawn from the findings
   e. Generalization of the study findings
   f. Implications of the findings for nursing
   g. Recommendations for further research
6. Introduction
7. theoretical and empirical or research
8. skimming, comprehending, and analyzing
9. identifying and understanding the steps of the research process
10. determining the value of the research report's content by examining the quality and completeness of the steps of the research process and the links among these steps

Types of Quantitative Research

1. a
2. b
3. b
4. d
5. a
6. c
7. a
8. b
9. c
10. b
11. c or d
12. a
13. b
14. a
15. c

EXERCISE 3: WEB-BASED INFORMATION AND RESOURCES

1. a. The National Human Genome Research Institute (NHGRI) is the name of the organization focused on human genome research in the US.
   b. The website for the institute is: https://www.genome.gov/
   c. The funding website of NHGRI is: https://www.genome.gov/12010633/overview-of-the-extramural-research-program/
   d. Genomic research began with the Human Genome Project (HGP).
2. a. The NINR website is: https://www.ninr.nih.gov/
   b. The "Research Funding Opportunities" are found on the following website: https://www.ninr.nih.gov/researchandfunding/fundingopportunities
   c. NINR Mission and Strategic Plan website: https://www.ninr.nih.gov/aboutninr/ninr-mission-and-strategic-plan
3. The website presenting the reports funded by the AHRQ is: https://www.ahrq.gov/research/findings/index.html
4. The website for the Centers for Disease Control and Prevention is: https://www.cdc.gov
5. Coronavirus Disease

EXERCISE 4: CONDUCTING CRITICAL APPRAISALS TO BUILD AN EVIDENCE-BASED PRACTICE

Type of Quantitative and/or Qualitative Research
1. d. (Because randomized controlled trials are usually considered experimental studies. However, c. (Quasi-experimental research could also be considered correct.)
2. f. (Grounded theory research method in which the goal is to develop a theory or framework about the care experience of patients with intravenous drug use/abuse-related endocarditis and how that concern is resolved or processed.)
3. c and g. (Greene and Ramos conducted a mixed methods study that included correlational quantitative and exploratory-descriptive qualitative methods.)

Type of Setting

1. b. Steffen et al. (2021, p. e204) reported the research setting for their study was health units that were "selected on the basis of the similarity of epidemiologic profile and health indicators in T2DM [Type 2 Diabetes Mellitus] and AH [arterial hypertension]." These health units allowed for controlled implementation of the intervention and measurement of study variables. However the heath units were clinical and not research focused.
2. a or b. Colwill et al., 2021, Participants section) reported their "study was conducted in the inpatient setting within a quaternary care medical center in the Midwest." Most qualitative studies are conducted in natural settings but the hospital setting might also be considered partially controlled.
3. a. Greene and Ramos (2021) reported the qualitative method of their study included simi-structured telephone interviews and the quantitative method included a secondary analysis of survey data. Both settings would be considered natural with phone interviews in the home and secondary analysis of participant survey data.

Type of Research Conducted (Applied or Basic)
1. a
2. a

CHAPTER 3—INTRODUCTION TO QUALITATIVE RESEARCH

EXERCISE 1: TERMS AND DEFINITIONS

General Terms

1. f
2. s
3. l
4. i
5. p
6. o
7. h
8. k
9. e
10. g
11. b
12. j
13. r
14. q
15. t
16. d
17. m
18. c
19. a
20. n

Definitions Related to Ethnography

1. d
2. f
3. g
4. b
5. c
6. e
7. a

Definitions in Your Own Words

1. Observation is gathering data by being in specific environments and situations and using all of your senses to notice and record details.
2. Coding is assigning a label to a key phrase or sentence in a transcript. The codes are synthesized into themes.
3. Researcher–participant relationship involves the communication and trust that connects the researcher and the participants. The relationship encourages or hinders the willingness of participants to share their perspectives.

EXERCISE 2: LINKING IDEAS

People and Their Contributions to Qualitative Research

1. d
2. a
3. c
4. b

Qualitative Research Methodology

1. dwell
2. native
3. field notes
4. saturation
5. probes

Approaches to Qualitative Research

1. G
2. E
3. P
4. E
5. EDQ
6. G
7. P
8. EDQ

EXERCISE 3: WEB-BASED INFORMATION AND RESOURCES

1. You may have found other journals that primarily publish qualitative research. The table includes some examples.

Journal Name	Publisher	URL
Qualitative Research	Sage	https://journals.sagepub.com/home/qrj (same for the following 2 Sage journals)
Qualitative Health Research	Sage	https://journals.sagepub.com/home/qrj
International Journal of Qualitative Methods	Sage	https://journals.sagepub.com/home/ijq
Qualitative Health Research	Emerald Insight	https://www.emerald.com/insight/publication/issn/1443-9883
American Journal of Qualitative Research	AJQR is sponsored and published by Center for Ethnic and Cultural Studies (CECS)	https://www.ajqr.org/home/about-journal
Ethnography	Sage	https://journals.sagepub.com/home/eth
European Journal of Qualitative Research in Psychotherapy	Open Journal System	http://www.ejqrp.org/index.php/ejqrp
Global Qualitative Nursing Research	Sage	https://us.sagepub.com/en-us/nam/journal/global-qualitative-nursing-research
International Journal of Qualitative Studies on Health and Well-Being	Taylor Francis Online	https://www.tandfonline.com/toc/zqhw20/current
Journal of Ethnographic & Qualitative Research	Cedarville University	https://www.jeqr.org/home

2.

Study Characteristic	Answer
Country in which the study was conducted.	Iran
Identify the qualitative approach conducted (phenomenology, grounded theory, exploratory-descriptive qualitative, ethnography research).	Phenomenology
Identify the human experience or topic of the study.	Moral distress of nurses who care for older adults in long term care facilities
Describe the sample, including the total number, number of males, number of females, average age, and average number of years of job experience. See Table 1.	9 participants, 4 males and 5 females $33.82(SD = 8.06)$ years $10.36(SD = 7.95)$ years
How were the data collected?	In-depth, semi-structured interviews were conducted with the nurses by one of the researchers with training in interview procedures. The interviews were checked by the first author.

3. a. One possible definition is "the study of people in their own environment through the use of methods such as participant observation and face-to-face interviewing." Another definition on the website is "first hand, detailed account of a given community or society attempts to get a comprehensive understanding of the circumstances of the people being studied."
   b. Cultural anthropologists

4. You may have selected one of the following websites or another that you may have found.
   https://podcasts.ox.ac.uk/keywords/qualitative-research
   https://player.fm/podcasts/Qualitative
   https://qualpage.com/2018/07/12/qualitative-podcasts-to-check-out/
   https://podcasts.apple.com/gb/podcast/ethnography-atelier-podcast/id1444653741
   https://www.wordsmatter-education.com/blog/podcast-43
   https://www.ncrm.ac.uk/resources/podcasts/
   https://www.podomatic.com/podcasts/aeraqrsig
   https://odum.unc.edu/datanight/

EXERCISE 4: CONDUCTING CRITICAL APPRAISALS TO BUILD AN EVIDENCE-BASED PRACTICE

1. Grounded theory using Strauss and Corbin's method (1998)

2. Yes, the outcome of grounded theory is a narrative describing social processes that may be accompanied by a diagram or model. Colwill et al. (2021, 3.1 The model) described their model in this way: "The model presented here is the integration of categories that emerged from the data and describes the core concept of cyclical life experiences of PWID [persons who inject drugs] who are hospitalized with endocarditis (Fig. 1). The model is made up of 2 inter-related cycles we called *The Person* and *The Healthcare System,* that exist within the cycle of *Society*. Endocarditis is the catalyst that initiates change and drives the process forward as the individual enters *The Healthcare System.* Expressions of hope and hopelessness co-exist with behaviors of the use/abuse cycle still present whether the individual was in *The Healthcare System* or *Society*. Quotations by the individuals are used to explicate the model."

3. Yes, the sections were clearly identified and well-written. Each section contained the content that a reader would expect to be in that section. The longest section was the Results section, which is common in qualitative study because the results are textual, instead of numerical.

4. The statement of research problem was identified as being a gap in the literature because no studies have described the perspectives of PWID and have developed endocarditis. Their experiences as they move in and out of the hospital was the primary focus.
   The researchers identified the the the aim (purpose) of the study to be developing a model to describe how PWID "interpret their lives as they move in and out of the hospital and society" (Colwill et al., 2021, 2. Methods).
   The study methodology was clearly identified in the title and described in the Methods section. The researchers stated they selected grounded theory because it was appropriate for developing theories and models.
   The initial review of the literature was limited which is common in grounded theory studies. The researchers identified the study by Bearnot et al. (2019) as describing the experiences of PWID when they encounter the health system. The findings of the Bearnot et al. (2019) study led to the current study. Colwill et al. (2021) wanted to better understand the needs of PWID. Additional studies and references are cited in the Discussion section of the article.
   There was no theoretical framework identified for the study, which is not uncommon in grounded theory studies.
   The single research question was "How do PWID hospitalized with endocarditis interpret their lives as they move in and out of the hospital and society?" (Colwill et al., 2021, 2. Methods).
   The methods were described in the study including how data were collected through interviews conducted with 11 participants selected through theoretical purposive sampling. The setting was an inpatient facility in the Midwest. The interviews were recorded, transcribed, and the data analyzed using the constant comparison method. The researchers described the coding processes that were used (open, axial, and selective coding). After 20 iterations of the model, the team felt they understood the themes and agreed on the core concept being PWID's cyclic life experiences.
   The results were presented as a model with the themes supported by participant quotations.

The <u>findings</u> were compared to previous studies, in some cases which supported the themes found by Colwill et al. (2021) and in other cases contrasted this study's results. The limitations were identified as being a small sample (as is common with qualitative studies) in one setting in one city and state. One of the implications for practice was the need for increased understanding of PWID that may lead to therapeutic communication and meeting the needs of this population more effectively. The need to reduce overt and perceived stigma of PWID was specifically identified as being needed. Colwill et al, (2021) noted that additional research was needed to understand the best ways to care for PWID.

5. Yes, the step of identifying a theoretical framework was missing. This is not uncommon in qualitative studies, especially grounded theory studies. If an appropriate theoretical framework is available, there may not be a need for a grounded theory study. Grounded theory studies are conducted to describe social processes and develop a theory or model.

6. Yes, the interviewers started the interview with the request: "Tell me what it is like being admitted to the hospital" (Colwill et al., 2021, Box 1). The study was designed to address the lack of knowledge about the perspectives of PWID who are hospitalized.

7. Yes, the grand tour question directly addressed the research question of how PWID interpret their lives when they are repeatedly hospitalized and then discharged.

8. Through close reading of the description of the analysis process, you will find that the model was developed with the data generated through the first eight interviews. Then three additional individuals were interviewed to confirm the model. The length of the interviews was not identified in the report. However, from the number and richness of the themes and supporting quotations, we can infer that the interviews were adequate in number and length.

9. The data analysis processes that were used were constant comparison with open, axial, and selective coding. These processes are consistent with Strauss and Corbin's (1998) grounded theory methods. These methods directly addressed the research problem, purpose, and research question. The interpretation of the analysis to produce a model was described in detail and readers can be confident in the study results.

10. The researchers described the analysis of the data in detail, including the use of memos. More is stated about the rigor of the study in section 4.1 Strengths and limitations. However, the researchers did not mention an audit trail, which is how analysis and interpretation decisions are usually documented. A method that is not stated, but may have occurred, would have been preparing minutes of their team meetings.

11. You may have selected any of the 3 overall themes and their subcomponents and provide an example of the supporting quotations. Here are examples, one from each theme.
    Theme: The person. "Individuals reported a loss of control to their addiction as Carlos described, "You are always chasing that high" (Colwill et al., 2021, 3.2.1.2. Loss of control).
    Theme: The healthcare system. " 'I do not want to do drugs. It was a second chance at life. They told me I would not last 10 hours. When they told me that, it changed my whole state on life and drugs itself" (Colwill et al., 2021, 3.2.2.1 Second chance).
    Theme: Society. "I've never had nobody, nobody to care for me. It's always been me by myself. (voice cracking)…"(Colwill et al., 2021, 3.2.3.2 Trauma and pain).

12. The researchers provided a thorough description of the analysis process. The processes used, the number of model iterations, and the richness of the findings indicate rigorous data analysis and interpretation.

Greene and Ramos (2021) Study

1. The qualitative data for the study were collected through 40 semi-structured telephone interviews that lasted about 20 minutes.

2. The data collection was adequate with a larger than normal sample for a qualitative study. Because the interviews were not lengthy, they did not produce as much data as longer interviews would have. With 40 interviews, however, adequate data were collected. The data were analyzed using descriptive thematic analysis. The researchers specified who analyzed the data initially and assigned codes. Other members of the team identified text blocks for each code and determined if additional codes were needed. The lead researchers (the authors) reconciled differences among the codes and identified sub-themes.

3. The key dimensions of trust in one's healthcare provider were identified as communication, caring, and competence. You only need to include one example, but here are examples for each of the dimensions. Communication: "A 38- year-old woman described the importance of her provider preparing her for cancer treatment: 'She made me feel comfortable every step of the way. She explained everything to me thoroughly and . . . told me what to expect. So there were no surprises as I was dealing with my treatment'" (Greene & Ramos, 2021, p. 1225). Caring: "A 53-year-old woman explained, 'I know that she's going to do her best to help me get through whatever is going on . . . She's going to just try to help me'" (Greene & Ramos, 2021, p. 1225). Competence: "Others described providers they trusted in the following ways: 'she knows what she's talking about' and 'he is very astute'" (Greene & Ramos, 2021, p. 1226).

CHAPTER 4—EXAMINING ETHICS IN NURSING RESEARCH

EXERCISE 1: TERMS AND DEFINITIONS

1. o
2. m
3. f
4. a
5. q
6. j
7. d
8. n
9. c
10. e

11. r
12. t
13. h
14. s
15. k
16. g
17. i
18. l
19. b
20. p

EXERCISE 2: LINKING IDEAS

1. a. Disclosure of essential study information to the subject
   b. Comprehension of this information by the subject
   c. Competency of the subject to give consent
   d. Voluntary consent by the subject to participate in the study
2. You might have identified any five of the following general information requirements of a study consent form.
   a. Purpose and procedures of the study
   b. Length of the subject's involvement
   c. Benefits and risks or discomforts
   d. Compensation, if any, for research-related injury

   e. Disclosure of alternative treatments if available
   f. Confidentiality of records
   g. Contact persons
   h. Right to refuse or withdraw without loss of benefit
3. diminished autonomy
4. institutional review boards (IRBs)
5. a. Exempt from review
   b. Expedited review
   c. Full review
6. Chairperson of the IRB
7. Breach of confidentiality. Raw data should not have participants' names included, but code numbers to maintain confidentiality. Only approved members of the research team should have access to raw data. Additionally, extra care should be taken to ensure confidentiality of sensitive information such as being able to spread Hepatis C to another person.
8. Full review
9. Common Rule
10. You may have selected any 3 of these possible answers:
    a. Fabrication of research results and recording or reporting fabricated results
    b. Falsification of research by manipulating research materials, equipment, or processes
    c. Falsification of research by changing, or omitting data or results
    d. Plagiarism by using another person's ideas, processes, results or words without giving proper credit
    e. Duplicate publication which is publishing a study in more than one journal without documenting the original publication
10. Yes, research misconduct is a current area of concern in nursing. Rationale may include recent plagiarism in published articles, research misconduct that led to a retraction in the journal of publication, or reports of misconduct from the Office of Research Integrity. A duplicate publication of the same study without citing previous publications of the study is a common type of misconduct in nursing and medicine. The need to always be vigilant to prevent or identify misconduct in nursing research is another possible answer.

Historical Events, Ethical Codes, and Regulations

1. b
2. a
3. d
4. c
5. a

6. c
7. d
8. b
9. b
10. a

Federal Regulations Influencing the Conduct of Research

1. b
2. a
3. b
4. c
5. a

Ethics of Published Studies

1. c
2. d
3. b
4. a

EXERCISE 3: WEB-BASED INFORMATION AND RESOURCES

1. The website for US DHHS is: https://www.hhs.gov/ohrp/regulations-and-policy/regulations/45-cfr-46/index.html
   The URL you identified may be slightly different depending on how you searched. Be sure that you found the Common Rule revised in 2018.
2. Pregnant women, human fetuses, and neonates involved in research
3. Website for the Belmont Report is: https://www.hhs.gov/ohrp/regulations-and-policy/belmont-report/read-the-belmont-report/index.html
4. 1974
5. 3 physicians, 0 nurses
6. Information, comprehension, voluntariness
7. Website for the ORI is: https://ori.hhs.gov/
8. When this key was prepared, there were 3 case summaries of research misconduct for 2021. When you answered this question, additional case summaries may be available.
   Lin- falsified, fabricated, and plagiarized data and text
   Wang- falsified data
   Yin- falsified and/or fabricated data and reporting research methods and statistics that were not performed
9. Website for Human Subjects research at the National Human Genome Research Institute is: https://www.genome.gov/about-genomics/policy-issues/Human-Subjects-Research-in-Genomics
10. Website for the FDA Clinical Trials and Human Subject Protection is: https://www.fda.gov/science-research/science-and-research-special-topics/clinical-trials-and-human-subject-protection

EXERCISE 4: CONDUCTING CRITICAL APPRAISALS TO BUILD AN EVIDENCE-BASED PRACTICE

1. Steffen et al. (2021) indicated their study was approved by the appropriate Research Ethics Committee. The research ethics committees in other countries have the same functions as institutional review boards (IRBs) in the U.S. The researchers noted that the study was designed to be compliant with two sets of Brazilian ethical standards for the protection of human subjects. Because the study involved an intervention for participants with cardiovascular risks, some IRBs would conduct a full review. However, other IRBs would evaluate the study as being appropriate for an expedited review because the intervention was designed to motivate behavioral change and did not involve a change in treatment or medication. The benefits of participation were not specified but can be inferred as the potential reduction in cardiovascular risk as indicated by improvements in the participants' HbA1c and blood pressure. The study posed little risk to the participants because of the nature of the intervention and the procedures that were implemented for randomization, scheduling, and obtaining informed consent. The confidentiality of the participants' information was protected by limiting access to the electronic files and scheduling system to persons who were recruiting participants. Informed consent was obtained ethically. To avoid coercion, participants who gave verbal consent received the consent document by mail and provided information about their participation. Only persons who signed the informed consent were included in the study. Children, patients who were illiterate, and patients with mental and behavioral diagnoses were excluded from the study. Therefore, there were no persons in the study who might have been more vulnerable to undue influence. The article does not include the content of the informed consent document, which is common. The inclusion criteria were justifiable based on the study's purpose and the intervention. Steffen et al. (2021) described the randomization and recruitment processes with adequate detail to determine they were conducted fairly. The researchers implemented a study that protected the autonomy and rights of the participants, followed ethical standards, and minimized harm and risk.

2. Colwill et al. (2021) indicated the study was approved by the hospital's IRB. The level of review was likely a full board review because the participants' addiction-related behaviors put them at higher risk if their identities were compromised during the study. Pseudonyms were used; however, Table 1 provided a demographic description of each participant by pseudonym. Nurses who cared for these patients might have known them well enough to link characteristics and participants quotations, threatening their confidentiality. Likely the IRB proposal included additional information about labeling and separating the recordings and transcripts from the signed consent forms or it would not have been approved. The benefits of the study were not stated, but inferred. Talking about their life experiences may have been helpful to the participants. The primary risks were the potential loss of confidentiality and becoming emotionally or psychologically upset during the interview. From the information provided, the rights of the participants appeared to be protected. The standards for ethical studies were maintained, except for a small potential for loss of confidentiality. Using summary variables about the sample in Table 1 would have been more appropriate.

3. Greene and Ramos (2021) reported their mixed methods study was approved by the IRBs of Urban Institute and Baruch College. The Urban Institute was the center that implemented the Health Reform Monitoring Survey (HRMS) and employed the second author. Baruch College was the employer of the first author. The level of IRB review for the study was most likely expedited. (It was not exempted because contact information was retained for the HRMS participants, at least for those who agreed to be contacted later for an interview.) There were no direct benefits to participants, but they knew they were contributing to efforts to improve healthcare. The risks were few because the methods were completing a survey and possibly being interviewed. The greatest risk was loss of confidentiality. The risk to confidentiality was minimized by 1) an independent survey company scheduling the interviews and interviewer being given only the telephone number and first name of the interviewee; and 2) the researchers stating that no identifying information was attached to the recordings or transcript files. For the interviews, verbal consent was obtained because the participants were interviewed by

telephone. To summarize, the Greene and Ramos (2021) study was conducted according to ethical standards and the rights of the human participants were protected.

CHAPTER 5—EXAMINING RESEARCH PROBLEMS, PURPOSES, AND HYPOTHESES

EXERCISE 1: TERMS AND DEFINITIONS
1. g
2. i
3. f
4. d
5. j
6. b
7. e
8. k
9. a
10. h
11. c

Types of Hypotheses
1. f
2. e
3. h
4. d
5. b
6. c
7. g
8. a

EXERCISE 2: LINKING IDEAS

Research Problem and Purpose
1. a. variables or concepts
   b. population
   c. setting
2. You might have identified any of the following or thought of another relevant reason:
   a. has an impact on or is applied in nursing practice
   b. expands previous research
   c. expands knowledge for nursing education and administration
   d. improves understanding of a problem by developing a model, framework, or theory
   e. adds knowledge to current nursing research priorities
   f. is related to health problems that affect a large number of people
   g. is related to health problems that have high morbidity and mortality rates.
3. a. researchers' expertise, which focuses on educational preparation, research previously conducted, and clinical experiences
   b. financial commitment
   c. adequate number of study participants
   d. Necessary facility and equipment are available

4. You might have identified any of the following agencies or organizations: National Institute for Nursing Research (NINR), Agency for Healthcare Research and Quality (AHRQ), *Healthy People 2030,* World Health Organization (WHO), American Association of Critical-Care Nurses (AACN), National Association of Neonatal Nurses, Oncology Nursing Society (ONS), or Society of Pediatric Nurses. You might have identified other national nursing agencies or professional organizations that have research priorities identified online or in publications.
5. significance and feasibility
6. concepts, population
7. qualitative study, exploratory-descriptive qualitative study, or ethnography
   Source: Mason, A., Salami, B., Salma, J., Yohani, S., Amin, M., Okeke-Ihejirika, P., & Ladha, T. (2021). Health information seeking among immigrant families in Western Canada. *Journal of Pediatric Nursing, 58*, 9-14. https://doi.org/10.1016/j.pedn.2020.11.009
8. outcomes study
   Source: Hernandez, J. M., Munyan, K., Thompson, K., Wilson, C., Arena, S., & Noack, D. (2021). Interprofessional education safe patient handling and mobility workshop for persons of size. *International Journal of Safe Patient Handling & Mobility, 11*(1), 6-15.
9. qualitative and quantitative
10. correlational quantitative study or quantitative study
    Source: Wahl, A. K., Osborne, R. H., Larsen, M. H., Andersen, M. H., Holter, I. A., & Borge, C. R. (2021). Exploring health literacy needs in chronic obstructive pulmonary disease (COPD): Associations between demographic, clinical variables, psychological well-being and health literacy. *Heart & Lung, 50*(3), 417-424. https://doi.org/10.1016/j.hrtlng.2021.02.007

Understanding Hypotheses

1. b, c, e, h
2. a, c, f, h
3. b, c, e, h
4. a, d, f, h
5. b, c, e, h
6. b, d, e, h
7. a, c, f, g
8. a, c, e, h
9. b, d, e, h
10. b, c, e, h

11. b, d, f, g
12. a, c, e, h
13. b, c, e, h
14. You could state the directional hypothesis in either of the following ways:
    a. Increased age, decreased family support, and decreased health status are related to decreased self-care abilities in nursing home residents.
    b. Decreased age, increased family support, and increased health status are related to increased self-care abilities in nursing home residents.
15. Patients with chronic low-back pain receiving low-back massage experience no difference in their perceptions of low-back pain from those receiving no massage.

Identifying Types of Study Variables

1. a
2. c
3. b
4. a
5. a or b
6. a
7. b
8. a
9. c
10. b
11. c
12. b
13. b
14. a or b
15. c

Understanding Study Variables

1. b
2. c
3. d
4. a
5. e
6. d
7. a
8. d
9. b
10. e

EXERCISE 3: WEB-BASED INFORMATION AND RESOURCES

1. The website is https://www.cdc.gov/
2. Yes. The website is https://www.cdc.gov/violenceprevention/childabuseandneglect/index.html
3. The website is https://www.cdc.gov/obesity/index.html
4. The website is https://www.cdc.gov/coronavirus/2019-ncov/vaccines
5. The website it: https://www.ons.org
6. The website is https://www.ninr.nih.gov/
7. The website is https://www.ninr.nih.gov/aboutninr/ninr-mission-and-strategic-plan
8. The website is https://www.diabetes.org

EXERCISE 4: CONDUCTING CRITICAL APPRAISALS TO BUILD AN EVIDENCE-BASED PRACTICE

Problem and Purpose

Steffen et al. (2021) Study

1. Research problem
   a. Significance of the problem: "Type 2 diabetes mellitus (T2DM) is a serious public health problem worldwide. When associated with a diagnosis of arterial hypertension (AH), T2DM has even higher morbidity and mortality, requiring increased efforts in its management. One of the main challenges in preventing, treating, and controlling T2DM and AH is strategizing with the person at the center of care, engaging patients and supporting patients' shared decision making—interventions in which primary care nurses play an important role" (Steffen et al., 2021, p. e204).
   b. Background of the problem: "Motivational interviewing (MI) is a collaborative style of communication. Clinical evidence has shown that MI strengthens the person's motivation and commitment to change behaviors in the interest of their health, on the basis of respect for their autonomy. ... In primary care environments, MI is an inexpensive and high-potential impact strategy that can be learned by different categories of health professionals and applied regardless of age, sex, or severity of the patient's health problem (Steffen et al., 2021, p. e204).
   c. Problem statement: "The prevailing reality is still that of epidemiologically alarming numbers of chronic conditions with standards of care that are generally inefficient, unsystematic, prescriptive, rushed, and with lack of dignity for the patient" (Steffen et al., 2021, p. e204).
2. Study purpose: "The aim of this study is to evaluate the effectiveness of MI in individual nursing consultations for the management of T2DM with AH in the context of primary health care" (Steffen et al., 2021, p. e204).
3. Yes, the problem and purpose are significant because of the increased morbidity and mortality rates for patients diagnosed with T2DM and AH. Another challenge is engaging patients in shared decision making to promote a healthy lifestyle, which is an important management role for nurses (see the Problem discussion in Question 1). The research purpose clearly addresses the identified problem.

4. Elements of the research purpose
   a. Variables: This study is a randomized controlled trial (RCT) that should focus on determining the effectiveness of an intervention on selected outcomes (Grove & Gray, 2023). The independent variable or intervention was clearly identified as MI provided in individual nursing consultations. The dependent variables were not included in the study purpose and were not clearly identified until the Measures section of the article (see p. e206). The main outcome was hemoglobin A1c (HbA1c) and the secondary outcome was blood pressure (BP).
   b. Population: Participants were individuals with T2DM and an associated diagnosis of AH.
   c. Settings: The purpose indicated that the study was done in the context of primary health care but the actual setting was identified in the Methods section as three health units from the large Brazilian Community Health Service Hospital Group.
5. The problem and purpose are feasible because (a) The authors have the educational credentials and clinical affiliations to complete the study as discussed in Chapter 1 of this study guide; (b) no financial support for the study was reported; (c) adequate study participants were available through selected health units in hospitals; (d) sites for training the nurses in MI intervention were available; (e) health agencies and personnel were supportive of data collection; and (f) access to a laboratory for determining HbA1c values, and BP equipment for measuring systolic and diastolic pressures were available.

Colwill et al. (2021) Study

1. Research problem
   a. Significance of the problem: "Hospital admissions for person(s) who inject drugs (PWID) with infective endocarditis have doubled over the last decade (Kadri et al., 2019; Weiss et al., 2020), and surgical intervention is needed to improve survival (Long & Koyfman, 2018). PWID with infective endocarditis (hereafter referred to as endocarditis) have poorer surgical outcomes (Hussain et al., 2017; Kim et al., 2016; Rabkin et al., 2012; Rudasill et al., 2019...) including need for reoperation due to post-surgical relapse. ... Some healthcare workers in the U.S. and abroad hold negative stereotypes of PWID, adversely affecting access to needed services" (Colwill et al., 2021, Introduction section).

b. Background of the problem: "Individuals perceive these negative stereotypes from healthcare workers as feelings of humiliation and lack of fairness and dignity in healthcare settings (Klingemann, 2017). This creates a situation in which PWID feel the need to hide their addiction from providers, further resulting in reduced access to care (Biancarelli et al., 2019). In a study that explored perception of care in both the inpatient and outpatient settings, researchers found that PWID with endocarditis identified stigma, physical and social co-morbidities, an expected return to abuse, and lack of care coordination as common experiences when interacting with the healthcare system (Bearnot et al., 2019)" (Colwill et al., 2021, Introduction section).

c. Problem statement: "Researchers have not exclusively explored the hospitalized patient perspective in this unique population of PWID with endocarditis as they await a treatment decision. We sought to address the gap in the literature, recognizing that these patients are a rich resource regarding their own complex needs" (Colwill et al., 2021, Introduction section).

2. Research purpose
   a. This study did not identify a specific purpose. However the study title might be considered the study purpose: "A grounded theory approach to the care experience of patients with intravenous drug use/abuse-related endocarditis."
   b. This study was clearly directed by a research question. "The research question for this study was: How do PWID hospitalized with endocarditis interpret their lives as they move in and out of the hospital and society? The aim of this study was to develop a model to describe these phenomena" (Colwill et al., 2021, Methods section). This study was directed by a clear, concise research question followed by an aim that further clarified the goal of the study. You might consider the aim as a study purpose but it is too incomplete to direct the study. The aim lacked study concepts, population, and setting.
   c. The purpose of this grounded theory study was to describe and interpret the lives of PWID hospitalized with endocarditis as they move in and out of the hospital and society.

3. Yes, the problem, purpose, and research question are significant because PWID infected with endocarditis have doubled over the last decade, often require surgery, and experience poor surgical outcomes (see the research problem in Question 1). PWID are negatively perceived by health professionals resulting in poor quality care and ultimately decreased access to care.

4. Colwill et al. (2021) identified the concepts, population, and setting in their research question.
   a. The research concepts studied included: interpret their lives, move in and out of the hospital and society.
   b. Population for the study was PWID with endocarditis.
   c. The setting for this study was a hospital.

5. The problem and purpose of this study were feasible because: (a) the researchers had educational (DNP, PhD) and clinical expertise (certified clinical nurse specialist and nurse practitioner) to conduct this study; (b) the authors reported no external funding for their study; (c) an adequate number of PWID with endocarditis were obtained from a quaternary care medical center in the Midwest; (d) data were collected through interviews in private patient rooms; and (e) Midwest medical center was supportive of the study.

Greene and Ramos (2021) Study

1. Research problem
   a. Significance of the problem: "Trusting one's physician has long been considered essential for an effective patient-physician relationship. … Fundamentally, trust in health providers is important to patients because patients turn to providers when they have a health problem that they are unable to independently address [14-16]. When seeking health care, patients are vulnerable, and need to rely on health providers' ability and commitment to address their health issues" (Greene & Ramos, 2021, p. 1222).
   b. Background of the problem: "Over the last 20 years, research has found that patients who report more trust in their physician and other health care providers are more engaged with their care [4], more likely to follow through on recommended care and medications [5-7], and often have better control of chronic conditions [8-10]. Trust in one's health provider is also related to better

health care utilization, including greater continuity with a provider, not delaying care, and keeping appointments" (Greene & Ramos, 2021, p. 1222).

"Recently, a working group of health care leaders and patient advocates in the United States have called for making health care related trust measures a standard part of patient experience evaluation [32]" (Greene & Ramos, 2021, p. 1223).

   c. Problem statement: "However, given the variation in how trust has previously been conceptualized and measured [33-35], it is important to better understand what patients believe builds their trust in healthcare providers" (Greene & Ramos, 2021, p. 1223).

2. Research purpose

   a. "This mixed methods study uses qualitative methods to identify the health provider behaviors that patients report build trust, and quantitative methods to test the robustness of the findings using a national survey in the United States" (Greene & Ramos, 2021, p. 1223).

   b. Yes, the purpose was clear and concise in presenting the focus of the qualitative method in this study. The quantitative component of the purpose focused more on testing robustness of the findings from the qualitative part of the study. The setting for the study was not identified.

3. Yes, the problem is significant because trust is essential to a quality patient-healthcare provider relationship. Trust encourages patients to seek care earlier, follow-through on recommended care initiatives, and have better health outcomes. This study purpose addresses the problem statement and identifies the focus of this mixed methods study.

4. Some but not all of the elements of a research purpose were identified.

   a. The research concept was health care provider behaviors that build trust. The quantitative part of the study was a secondary analysis of data from the Health Reform Monitoring Survey (HRMS) that was correlated with the provider trust building behaviors identified in the qualitative part of the study (see Table 2, p. 1224).

   b. The population for the qualitative component of this study was individuals interviewed regarding their trust in healthcare providers. The population for

the quantitative component of the study was identified as participants in the US who completed the national HRMS.

   c. The qualitative interviews were conducted by phone so the setting was natural, probably the participant's home. Natural settings, such as homes or clinics, are usually used for a national survey, such as the HRMS.

5. The problem and purpose of this study were feasible because (a) the researchers have the expertise to conduct this study as indicated by their positions as a professor in School of Public Health and a position in a Health Policy Center; (b) the study was funded by the Robert Wood Johnson Foundation, a quality organization; (c) adequate participants were available and consented to participant in the telephone interviews; and (d) secondary data analysis was conducted using data from the large, national HRMS.

Objectives, Questions, and Hypotheses

Steffen et al. (2021) Study

1. Steffen et al. (2021) stated no objectives, questions, or hypotheses to direct their study.

2. No, because a RCT is an experimental study that should involve the testing of hypotheses. The lack of hypotheses in this study resulted in an unclear link between the purpose and the study methods. In addition, the Results section would have been more clearly organized and understandable if linked to hypotheses. Hypotheses also provide direction for the interpretations of findings and the linking of this study's findings to those of previous studies (Grove & Gray, 2023).

Colwill et al. (2021) Study

1. As discussed earlier, a research question was used to direct the conduct of this study. "The research question for this study was: How do PWID hospitalized with endocarditis interpret their lives as they move in and out of the hospital and society?"(Colwill et al., 2021, Methods section). In addition, an aim was developed to identify the proposed outcome of the study. "The aim of this study was to develop a model to describe these phenomena" (Colwill et al., 2021, Methods section).

2. Yes, this research question was appropriately for this grounded theory study and provided clear direction for conducting the study. The aim also clarified the proposed outcome for the study.

Greene and Ramos (2021) Study

1. Greene and Ramos (2021, p. 1222) stated the following objective in their abstract: "Objective: Patient trust in health care providers is associated with better health behaviors and utilization, yet provider trust has not been consistently conceptualized." However, this objective really is more typical of a problem statement and does not direct the conduct of this study (Grove & Gray, 2023). No specific objectives, questions or hypotheses were reported to direct this study. Therefore, you can assume this study is directed by the research purpose.

2. Often research questions or objectives are used to provide direction for the qualitative and quantitative methods of a mixed methods study. However, they are not essential and the purpose of this study does identify the focus of both the qualitative and quantitative parts of this study so is adequate to direct the study.

Study Variables and Concepts

Steffen et al. (2021) Study

The key study variables in quasi-experimental and experimental studies are identified in the study hypotheses. However, this study did not identify hypotheses.

Variable	Type of variable
Motivational interviewing (MI)	Independent variable
Hemoglobin A1c (HbA1c)	Dependent variable
Blood pressure (BP)	Dependent variable

a. Conceptual definition of MI intervention: "Motivational interviewing (MI) is a collaborative style of communication. Clinical evidence has shown that MI strengthens the person's motivation and commitment to change behaviors in the interest of their health, on the basis of respect for their autonomy" (Steffen et al., 2021, p. e204).

b. Operational definition of MI intervention: "The test/MI group received 2 MI-based nursing consultation sessions lasting 30 – 50 minutes and conducted monthly by nurses

who received 20 hours of training in the use of MI" (Steffen et al. (2021, p. e205). The details of the MI intervention are described and critically appraised in Chapter 8 Clarifying Quantitative Research Design of this study guide.

3. Yes, the conceptual and operational definitions for the MI were appropriate and clearly expressed in this study. The conceptual definition was expressed in the Introduction section and had a strong link to the operational definition in the Methods section. The definitions are easy for the readers to identify and understand. However, Steffen et al. (2021) did not identify a study framework and the conceptual definition had to be abstracted from the review of literature. Thus, the link of the conceptual definition to nursing theory and knowledge is missing.

4. The sociodemographic and health history characteristics of the patients in the usual care and test/MI groups are presented in Table 1 (see p. e207). Therefore, the demographic variables included: sex (gender), age, race/ethnicity, lives alone, education level, marital status, per capita income, AH diagnosis time and years, T2DM diagnosis time and years, cardiovascular disease (CVD) family history, associated diseases, polypharmacy, depression symptoms, smoking, alcohol consumption, and time of physical exercise.

5. The extraneous variables were depression measured by the Beck Depression Inventory and adherence measured by the Martin-Bayarre-Grade Questionnaire. Depression and adherence were thought to have confounding effect on the outcomes, HbA1c and BP, and could bias the study findings.

Greene and Ramos (2021) Study

1. Study concept is healthcare provider behaviors that build trust
   The description and critical appraisal of the steps in this mixed methods study are detailed in Chapter 14.

2. The demographic variables included in this study were gender, age, education, income, race/ethnicity, and health insurance. The sample characteristics for the interview and survey participants are presented in Table 1 (see p. 1223).

CHAPTER 6—UNDERSTANDING AND CRITICALLY APPRAISING THE LITERATURE REVIEW

EXERCISE 1: TERMS AND DEFINITIONS

1.	l	9.	k
2.	a	10.	j
3.	m	11.	b
4.	o	12.	p
5.	h	13.	f
6.	i	14.	e
7.	c	15.	g
8.	d	16.	n

EXERCISE 2: LINKING IDEAS

Examples of Main Ideas from the Chapter

1. (1) relevant; (2) critically appraising; (3) synthesizing; (4) accurate, complete
2. known, not known
3. theoretical, scientific or empirical
4. five
5. quantitative
6. periodical
7. peer-reviewed
8. purpose
9. You may have included any of the following: valid, appropriate, current, relevant, accurate, without bias, and quality. There may be others.
10. summary table or conceptual map

Theoretical and Empirical Sources

1.	T	6.	E
2.	E	7.	T
3.	E	8.	E
4.	E	9.	T
5.	T	10.	E

Primary and Secondary Sources

1.	S	6.	P
2.	P	7.	P
3.	P	8.	S
4.	S	9.	P
5.	P	10.	P

EXERCISE 3: WEB-BASED INFORMATION AND RESOURCES

1. https://www.ncbi.nlm.nih.gov/pmc/articles/PMC6862708/
2. a. Defining your main topic
   b. Searching the literature
   c. Analyzing your results
   d. Writing
   e. Reflecting on your writing
3. https://www.nlm.nih.gov/
4. https://www.nlm.nih.gov/portals/healthcare.html
5. https://www.ncbi.nlm.nih.gov/nlmcatalog/
6. https://owl.purdue.edu/owl/purdue_owl.html
7. a. Introduction
   b. Body
   c. Conclusion
8. You may have identified chronological, thematic, methodological, or theoretical. Here are descriptions of these organizing strategies. Compare your answer to the answer for the one you selected.
   Chronological—begin with the older sources, moving to more recent sources to show the development of the topic over time.
   Thematic—you identified a central idea throughout your review of the literature. You can organize the review by different aspects of that central idea.
   Methodological—you can describe the quantitative studies separately, followed by the qualitative studies and mixed methods studies. In a similar way, you may organize the review by descriptive studies, correlational studies, quasi-experimental, and experimental studies.
   Theoretical—during the review, you have identified the primary theoretical perspectives on your topic and you organize your sources by these perspectives.
9. Al-Shamaly (2021) used the thematic approach to organizing the literature review. The first paragraph identified the research done about different perspectives and aspects of caring in the ICU. The second paragraph included nursing workforce issues, such practices and communication. The third paragraph describes the research problem and statement.

EXERCISE 4: CONDUCTING CRITICAL APPRAISALS TO BUILD AN EVIDENCE-BASED PRACTICE

Steffen et al. (2021)

1. The first paragraph described the poor health outcomes associated with T2DM and AH and the challenge of keeping the patient at the center of care. Motivational interviewing was the main idea of the second paragraph. The third paragraph concluded that findings of recent studies were promising but not applied in practice. As a result, care of persons with T2DM and AH was "generally inefficient, unsystematic,

prescriptive, rushed, and with lack of dignity for the patient" (Steffen et al., 2021, e204). Essentially, the first three paragraphs included the clinical problem, the problem significance, the background, and the problem statement.

2. Welch et al. (2010) described the results of a meta-analysis. You may have also noticed that Lundahl and Burke (2009) reported a practice friendly review of four meta-analyses.

3. Steinberg and Miller (2015) is a book about motivational interviewing. Chen et al. (2012) is an older nursing study (randomized control trial) of the effects of motivational interviewing on outcomes of persons with T2DM. Moyers et al. (2007) is a manual about scales that measure intervention fidelity of motivational interviewing. You might describe it as an electronic book or a PDF file.

Colwill et al. (2021)

1. The references were current because 23 of 25 (92%) were published in the past 10 years and 17 of 25 (68%) were published in the past 5 years.

2. DiMaio et al. (2009) addressed the ethical challenges faced by surgeons who perform aortic valve replacement for persons with D with infective endocarditis. The second, Strauss and Corbin (1998), is one of the classic references for grounded theory research.

3. One, Dion (2019) was the only reference published in a nursing journal.

4. Physicians; you might have also answered cardiologists or surgeons. The reasons for using medical references include that nursing researchers and clinicians had not written about the clinical problem nor identified the unique needs of this population. The clinical problem was medical in nature and required surgical intervention, Therefore, more physicians and medical researchers had published on the topic.

5. The quality of the literature cited in the paper is high because the sources are from peer-reviewed journals and were primary sources. Several of the cited studies reported outcomes of surgical intervention for PWID with infective endocarditis, which was an inclusion criterion for the study sample. Several references addressed addiction and the experiences of persons dealing with addictions. Other references supported the study methodology. The references of the Colwill et al. (2021) report were high quality and relevant.

Greene & Ramos (2021)

1. The references cited by Greene and Ramos (2021) were not current with only 33 of 51(64%) published in the past 10 years and 16 (31%) published in the past 5 years.

2. You might have identified any of the following: Anderson and Dedrick (1990); Thom et al. (2004); Egede and Ellis (2008); Hall et al. (2002); Dugan et al. (2005); Leisen and Hyman (2005); or Thom et al. (1999).

3. Trust

4. The studies and other references cited by Greene and Ramos (2021) in the Introduction may have been critically appraised, but the appraisal was not reported. However, the findings of the studies were compared and well synthesized. One example is this sentence: "Over the last 20 years, research has found that patients who report more trust in their physician and other health care providers are more engaged with their care [4], more likely to follow through on recommended care and medications [5–7], and often have better control of chronic conditions [8–10]" (Greene & Ramos, 2021, p. 1222).

5. The review of the literature was only five paragraphs long. Each paragraph had a clear focus and conclusion. There was no summary. However, Greene and Ramos (2021) identified what was known as being the importance of the concept of trust and the conflicting results of studies. What was not known was the patient's perspective of what builds trust in a provider. "Given the variation in how trust has previously been conceptualized and measured [33–35], it is important to better understand what patients believe builds their trust in health care providers" (Greene & Ramos, 2021, p. 1223). The researchers linked the study purpose and methods to this gap in knowledge.

CHAPTER 7—UNDERSTANDING THEORY AND RESEARCH FRAMEWORKS

EXERCISE 1: TERMS AND DEFINITIONS

1. j
2. h
3. e
4. b
5. k
6. c
7. i
8. a
9. f
10. g
11. l
12. m
13. d

Types of Theories

1. d
2. a
3. b
4. f
5. c
6. e

EXERCISE 2: LINKING IDEAS

Key Theoretical Ideas

1. statements
2. variable
3. propositions or relational statements
4. hypotheses
5. Orem
6. nursing intellectual capital
7. Research framework
8. Conceptual definitions are abstract, comprehensive definitions based on theory. Operational definitions are narrower and indicate how the variable will be measured, implemented, or observed in the specific study.
9. Grand nursing theories are abstract conceptual models that describe nursing. Middle range theories are less abstract and focus on a specific phenomenon or situation in practice. The example of a grand nursing theory may be any of the theories listed in Table 7.3 or another grand theory identified by searching online. The example of a middle range theory may be any of the theories listed in Table 7.4 or another middle range nursing theory identified by searching online.
10. Scientific theories have been refined and validated by a large body of research. Most scientific theories describe physiological and pathophysiological processes. Tentative theories are newly proposed and have limited research evidence to support them. Tentative theories may describe a new phenomenon or pull together separate relationships that have some research support.

Levels of Abstraction

Construct (*highest*)
Concept
Variable
Operational definition (*lowest*)

Elements of Theory

1. Heart Efficacy, Cardiac Output, Urinary Tract Output, and Blood Pressure
2. relationships between the concepts, also called statements or propositions
3. research framework

Examples of Frameworks

1. h
2. b
3. g
4. e
5. c
6. f
7. d
8. a

Example of Grand Theory Used in a Study

1. Roy's Adaptation Model (RAM)
2. a. Alzheimer's disease
   b. person's response
   c. Cognitive Stimulation Therapy
3. Coping and Adaptation Processing Scale

EXERCISE 3: WEB-BASED INFORMATION AND RESOURCES

1. There are likely other websites, but here are three possible answers.
   https://nursing-theory.org/nursing-theorists/Katharine-Kolcaba.php
   https://nursology.net/nurse-theories/kolcabas-comfort-theory/
   https://currentnursing.com/nursing_theory/comfort_theory_Kathy_Kolcaba.html
2. a. relief, b. ease, and c. transcendence
3. Possible websites for each of the theories. You may have found other websites. Several of the websites below are articles published about the theory.

Theory	Theorists	Website
Caring	Swanson	https://pmhealthnp.com/kristen-swanson-theory-of-caring-and-healing/ https://connect.springerpub.com/content/sgrcn/24/1/6 http://lormacollegesnursinginformatics2018.blogspot.com/2018/07/swanson-kristens-theory-theory-of-caring.html https://onlinelibrary.wiley.com/doi/abs/10.1111/j.1471-6712.2008.00647.x
Heat stress	Byrne & Ludington-Hoe	https://www.cdc.gov/nora/councils/hcsa/pdfs/26-Byrne-508.pdf

Theory	Theorists	Website
Nursing intellectual capital	Covell	https://ojin.nursingworld.org/MainMenuCategories/ ANAMarketplace/ANAPeriodicals/OJIN/TableofContents/Vol-18-2013/No2-May-2013/Nursing-Intellectual-Capital-Theory.html https://pubmed.ncbi.nlm.nih.gov/23758420/
Self-care in chronic illness	Riegel et al.	https://www.ncbi.nlm.nih.gov/pmc/articles/PMC6686959/ https://pubmed.ncbi.nlm.nih.gov/22739426/ https://nursology.net/nurse-theories/theory-of-self-care-of-chronic-illness/
Self-transcendence	Reed	https://www.tandfonline.com/doi/abs/10.3109/01612849609049920 https://journals.sagepub.com/doi/abs/10.1177/01939450122045492 https://psycnet.apa.org/record/1991-27391-001
Transitions	Meleis	https://pubmed.ncbi.nlm.nih.gov/16313379/ https://sigma.nursingrepository.org/handle/10755/243548 https://psycnet.apa.org/record/1994-46541-001 https://www.nursing.upenn.edu/live/files/552-transitions-theory
Uncertainty in illness	Mishel	https://jag.journalagent.com/phd/pdfs/PHD-44365-CASE_REPORT-TAS_BORA[A].pdf https://nursology.net/nurse-theories/mishels-uncertainty-in-illness-theory/ https://clinicaltrials.gov/ct2/show/NCT03431155
Unpleasant symptoms	Lenz	https://www.redalySc.org/journal/1452/145254388001/html/ https://pubmed.ncbi.nlm.nih.gov/9055027/ https://connect.springerpub.com/content/book/978-0-8261-9552-4/part/part02/chapter/ch08

4. You may have identified other concepts but these are possible answers for each theory in Table 7.4.

Theory	Theorists	Concepts
Caring	Swanson	Maintaining belief, Knowing, Being With, Doing For, Enabling, Client-Wellbeing
Heat stress	Byrne & Ludington-Hoe	Environmental heat stress, Cognizance of Environmental Factors, Modifications to Physical Factors, Responsiveness to Situational Factors, Personal heat stress, Situational heat stress
Nursing intellectual capital	Covell	Intellectual capital, Human capital, Structural capital, Relational capital, Capital investment,
Self-care in chronic illness	Riegel et al.	Self-care maintenance, Self-care monitoring, Self-care management,
Self-transcendence	Reed	Transcendence, Human development, End-of-life, Vulnerability, Well-being, Nurse-patient interaction
Transitions	Meleis	Transitions, Coping with change, Mastery of change, Disruptions, Change triggers, Critical points
Uncertainty in illness	Mishel	Stimuli frame, Cognitive capacities, Structure providers, Inference illusion, Danger, Opportunity, Coping, Adaptation, Danger, Opportunity
Unpleasant symptoms	Lenz	Symptoms, Influencing factors (Physiological, Psychological, Situational), Performance outcomes, Intensity, Timing, Distress

EXERCISE 4: CONDUCTING CRITICAL APPRAISALS TO BUILD AN EVIDENCE-BASED PRACTICE

Steffen et al. (2021) Critical Appraisal

1. Severity of the chronic condition, patient's self-management capabilities based on the Chronic Care Model

2. Inclusion criteria: "Study participants were individuals with T2DM [type 2 diabetes mellitus] and an associated diagnosis of AH, were registered in the health units established as the research settings, and were with Risk Strata 3 and 4" (Steffen et al., 2021, e204).

3. http://www.ihi.org/resources/Pages/Changes/ ChangestoImproveChronicCare.aspx Other websites may be found that have diagrams of the Chronic Care Model.

4. Answer could include any of the following: Community, Health System, Self-Management Support, Delivery System Design, Decision Support, Clinical Information System, Informed Activated Patient, Productive Interactions, Prepared Practice Team, Improved Outcomes.

5. The intervention of motivational interviewing was a component of *productive interactions* between the patient and provider aimed at increasing the *activation of the patient*. The nurses who implemented the motivational interviewing were member of the *prepared practice team*. The *improved outcomes* from the model were the study's dependent variables of HbA1c and blood pressure readings.

6. The researchers could have provided a description of all the components of the model or at least those relevant to the study as described in the previous answer. In the Discussion section, they could have identified how the evidence for improved outcomes using motivational interviewing supports these relationships within the model.

Colwill et al. (2021) Critical Appraisal

1. Relationships, Fear, Unmet needs, Second-class citizen, Trauma/pain

2. Want to die, Loss of control, Withdrawal

3. The quotations you selected as supporting a concept may be different than these examples. *Want to die*: Sarah said "curl up in a ball and die." Matt said, "I will be at peace once I am dead." *Loss of control:* Sarah said, "I was upset and mad and did not know what to do." Phil said, "It spirals out of control." *Withdrawal:* Sarah said, "you get high and you feel good." Tanya said, "It makes you sick if you take and makes you sick if you don't take it."

4. Second chance, Desire to live, Locus of control

5. Cyclic life experiences

6. Meleis' transition theory

7. The model emerged from participants' experiences, making it a substantive theory, with relevance for practice. The researchers note that it is a person-centered model. The model is also comprehensive with constructs, concepts, and processes. Relationships among the concepts are implied by their positions in the model, but not made explicit. For example, the person is inside society and the concepts related to person are shown as arrows that affect each other. The model is complex and fluid, which is a strength for practice but may be a weakness for research. Researchers would likely to use a component of the model as the framework for a study. For example, a quantitative researcher might compare the hope or desire to change of persons who inject drugs with endocarditis outside and inside the healthcare system to answer the question of whether entry into the healthcare system increases the desire to change.

Green and Ramos (2021) Critical Appraisal

1. Your answer could be the Wake Forest Physician Trust Scale, Trust in Physician Scale, Trust in Oncologist Scale (TiOS; Hillen et al., 2013), or Health Care Relationship Trust Scale (Bova et al., 2012).

2. For the Wake Forest Physician Trust Scale and Trust in Physician Scale, the conceptual definition is that trust is the patient's perception of the provider's fidelity, technical competence, confidentiality, and honesty. For the TiOS (Hillen et al., 2013), trust is the patient's perception of physician caring, fidelity, technical competence, confidentiality, and honesty. For the Health Care Relationship Trust Scale, trust is the patient's perception of the provider's interpersonal connection, respectful communication, and professional partnering.

3. Communication, caring, and competence. Trust is the patient's perception of the provider's communication, caring, and competence.

4. The competence-related items had the strongest correlations with trust.

5. Green and Ramos could have linked their findings to existing theories of communication, interpersonal relationships, or technical competence. They could have also linked their findings to nursing theories such as King's theory of goal attainment (mutually agreed-upon goals).

CHAPTER 8—CLARIFYING QUANTITATIVE RESEARCH DESIGNS

EXERCISE 1: TERMS AND DEFINITIONS

Understanding Common Design Terms

1.	j	10.	k
2.	p	11.	l
3.	a	12.	g
4.	n	13.	m
5.	f	14.	i
6.	q	15.	h
7.	d	16.	o
8.	e	17.	c
9.	b		

Design Validity Terms

Types of Design Validity

1. b
2. d
3. a
4. c

Threats to Design Validity

1.	j	8.	k
2.	c	9.	d
3.	n	10.	b
4.	i	11.	g
5.	m	12.	h
6.	a	13.	e
7.	f	14.	l

EXERCISE 2: LINKING IDEAS

1. causality
2. intervention
3. control
4. probability
5. prospective
6. design validity
7. predictive correlational design
8. treatment, intervention, or experimental group; control or comparison group
9. intervention fidelity
10. control
11. comparative descriptive
12. You might have listed any three of the following elements:
    a. The study includes a treatment or intervention.
    b. The experimental or treatment group receives the study intervention.

c. The intervention is manipulated by the researchers to create an outcome or effect.
    d. The study usually includes a control or comparison group.
    e. The extraneous variables are controlled as much as possible to reduce their influence on study findings.
    f. The study participants should be randomly assigned to either the intervention or control group.
    g. The study is strengthened if the study participants are randomly selected for the study.
13. The sample was too small or the study had inadequate power to find a relationship that may have existed.
14. Attrition
15. statistical conclusion

Determining Types of Design Validity in Studies

1.	b	6.	c
2.	d	7.	c
3.	a	8.	a
4.	c.	9.	d
5.	b	10.	a

Control and Designs for Nursing Studies

You may have worded your rationale and strengths differently but you should have included these key points.

1. **Design:** Quasi-experimental post-test-only design with comparison group
   Rationale: The sample was selected non-randomly because it was children undergoing a surgical procedure in one hospital. Selection was also dependent on the day of the week the surgery was scheduled. There was an intervention, the animated program on the computer. This study included a comparison group because participants were not randomly assigned.
   Study strengths: You should have included at least one of the following strengths. The intervention was delivered consistently, which was a study strength. The FACES rating scale is a well-established valid and reliable method for measuring acute pain in children. The age of the children was controlled, as was the setting for the study. The groups were equal in size.

2. **Design:** Descriptive correlational study
   Rationale: The purpose of the study was to examine relationships (correlations) among the variables of hours of sleep, stress level, anxiety

level, and depression in first-time mothers. The focus was not on predicting one variable based on the values of the other variables, so it was not a predictive correlational study.

Strengths: Limiting the sample to first-time mothers in the first month following the birth of their child was a way of controlling extraneous variables. Data collection occurred at one point in time so the study had no attrition of participants and no threats to history. The measurement methods in this study are unknown but need to be reliable and valid. Correlational studies have less control than quasi-experimental studies because the population is studied without manipulation in a natural setting.

3. **Design:** Quasi-experimental pretest and post-test design with control group

   Rationale: The intervention was the vitamins given to the treatment group. Infants were randomly assigned to groups. Weight was the outcome variable and it was measured at the beginning and end of the study. It was not an experimental design because the infants were in their homes during the study and other factors were not controlled such as time of day the vitamins were given or the type of formula may have varied among the infants.

   Strengths: The sample size was determined by power analysis. Although a non-random sample, the infants were randomly assigned to groups. The infants were the same age at the beginning of the study and had the same diagnosis. Data collection was controlled with the pretest being done prior to implementing the vitamin intervention and the post-test was conducted at 8 months of age. The intervention of vitamins was controlled by using a detailed protocol for implementation.

4. **Design:** Comparative descriptive design

   Rationale: The non-random sample were recruited from three different centers, but the researcher did not implement an intervention that was controlled. There was no indication that the same number of women was recruited from each center. The women were not randomly assigned to the centers.

   Strengths: The stage of cancer and the type of medical treatment (radiation) were controlled so that the sample was more homogenous. The homogenous sample reduced the likelihood that differences in the outcomes were due to the extraneous factors of cancer and treatment type. The instruments used were reported to be valid and reliable for this population.

5. **Design:** Randomized controlled trial (RCT)

   Rationale: The study was an RCT because of the controls that were implemented. Blinding was used to decrease social desirability and experimenter expectancy. The large sample was randomly assigned to the control and intervention groups. The study was conducted in multiple sites. The intervention was manipulated in a controlled way to ensure the right participants got the medication and that the medication was delivered accurately at the right time, right dose, and right route.

   Strengths: Measurement of blood pressure (BP) was controlled to ensure precise and accurate readings. Also, the implementation of the drug treatment for the intervention and control groups was controlled. Other strengths include blinding, large sample, random assignment, diverse locations, and safety precautions.

EXERCISE 3: WEB-BASED INFORMATION AND RESOURCES

1. CONsolidated Standards for Reporting Trials (CONSORT).
   The CONSORT website is: http://www.consort-statement.org/
2. 2018
3. https://www.nih.gov/grants-funding
   32 billion dollars
4. https://www.nih.gov/research-training
5. https://www.nih.gov/research-training/medical-research-initiatives
6. Several answers could be correct for this question. You may have identified one of these or you may have another answer. Discuss your answer with one of your fellow students to think more deeply about appropriate designs for this emerging health problems.
   Because what we know about post-acute sequelae of COVID (PASC) is limited, descriptive study designs may be what is needed first. Simple descriptive designs would be appropriate to describe the incidence, progression, and resolution of COVID long-term effects. Comparative descriptive designs would be appropriate to compare the incidence, symptoms, and resolution of COVID's long-term effects among existing groups, such as males and females or persons of different races and ethnicities, of different age groups, or different parts of the country.
   Correlational designs would be helpful to understand the relationships among variables

such as length of acute illnesses, days of hospitalization and ventilator use, and persons of different ages. You could design descriptive correlational studies or you could implement a predictive correlational design to predict the length of recovery from COVID using personal characteristics, medical history, symptoms, and treatments. As more is known about persons with PASC, intervention studies implementing new treatments or medications could be designed. Intervention studies include quasi-experimental and experimental designs.

7. https://clinicaltrials.gov/ct2/results?cond=Type+2+diabetes&term=NCT03729323&cntry=BR&state=&city=&dist
RCT is completed

EXERCISE 4: CONDUCTING CRITICAL APPRAISALS TO BUILD AN EVIDENCE-BASED PRACTICE

Steffen et al. (2021) Critical Appraisal

1. Double-blind parallel group randomized clinical trial (RCT)

2. a. Each participant in the treatment/intervention group received 2 motivational-interviewing sessions (30-50 minutes long) that were delivered approximately a month apart.
   b. Eight nurses delivered the intervention.
   c. To be selected to deliver the intervention, the nurses met the criteria of having specialized in public health and had 5 or more years of experience in primary care.
   d. The selected nurses were trained by a PhD-prepared psychologist with experience in motivational interviewing. The training included didactic and experiential components and lasted for 20 hours.
   e. Before and after the training, the nurses completed the following instruments: 1) Importance and Confidence Ruler for using MI; 2) Conversational Interview Exercise; 3) Helpful Responses Questionnaire; and 4) Motivational Interviewing Skills Code. These tools assessed perceived importance of MI, confidence in using MI, and mastery of initial basic skills in using MI.
   f. The fidelity of the MI intervention was strengthened by the selection of the nurses and their training. Their proficiency in delivering the intervention was assessed after the training. However, the fidelity would have been strengthened by the trainer observing each nurse delivering the intervention to a participant at the beginning, middle, and near the end of the study.

3. Yes, the study had a comparison or control group. Steffen et al. (2021) stated that the study had a test/MI group and a usual-care group. The researchers described the process by which potential participants who were eligible for the study were randomized to groups and a flow chart was shown in Figure 1. Individuals who were not the researchers identified potential participants, randomized them to groups, contacted them to determine whether they met the inclusion/exclusion criteria, and scheduled them for appointments.

4. You may have identified others but here are some possible design validity strengths.
Random assignment to groups supports internal design validity.
Data collectors were blinded to group assignment, which supports construct design validity.
Standard laboratory test for HgA1c and BP measurement are appropriate measurements for physiological variables, which strengthens the construct design validity.
Low attrition rate (7.9%) supports the internal design validity as does the attrition being similar between the treatment and usual care group (7% treatment group to 9% usual care group).
No indication of maturation or history so threats to internal validity were avoided.
The researchers used conservative approach of analyzing data of those who completed the study and those who left the study, called intent to treat, which supports the statistical analysis design validity.
Intervention was similar in time and scheduling as usual care, which supports external design validity.
Low refusal rate (7.8%) supports external design validity.

5. You may have identified others but here are some possible answers.
Threats to statistical conclusion design validity: No assessment of intervention fidelity during the study, smaller sample than was planned (low statistical power related to HbA1c), possible extraneous variables in the setting, and no information provided about the accreditation of the laboratory that analyzed the blood specimens for the HgA1c.

Each variable was measured with one operation, which is a possible threat to construct design validity. The researchers included participants regardless of whether their baseline HbA1c levels were within the therapeutic target, which is a threat to internal design validity regarding participant selection.

Greene and Ramos (2021) Study

1. Descriptive correlational
2. No, the design of the quantitative component of the study was not identified. You can infer from the text and the correlational values in Table 2 that the focus was on examining relationships, which is the purpose of descriptive correlational studies. The secondary analysis of the data from the Health Reform Monitoring Survey was conducted to "examine the relationship between trust and key components of trust identified in the qualitative component" (Greene & Ramos, 2021, p. 1223).
3. The Health Reform Monitoring Survey was designed to assess the impact of the Affordable Care Act. The data from the 2019 survey were used for this study. The data were collected from "Ipsos' internet panel that is representative of English and Spanish speakers aged 18-64 in the United States" (Greene & Ramos, 2021, p, 1224). The desired participants had a usual healthcare provider *(n* = 6392).
4. You may have identified other answers but here are some design validity strengths of the Greene and Ramos study.
   a. The sample was a nationally-representative sample that increased internal validity.
   b. Participants were diverse for race/ethnicity and range of incomes, increasing external validity.
   c. Study had a very large sample with strong statistical power, which strengthened the statistical conclusion validity.
   d. No reported attrition or evidence of history and maturation, which strengthened the internal validity.
5. Threats to the design validity of the Greene and Ramos (2021) study include:
   a. No reliability information was provided about the survey questions, threatening statistical conclusion design validity.
   b. Researchers identified that the conceptual and operational definitions of trust were unclear. Although the qualitative study component did provide a model of trust, the survey questions may not have measured exactly what was intended, which was a threat to construct design validity.

c. Each aspect of trust was measured by 1 or 2 survey questions, which was a mono-operation bias that threatens construct design validity.

CHAPTER 9—EXAMINING POPULATIONS AND SAMPLE IN RESEARCH

EXERCISE 1: TERMS AND DEFINITIONS
1. j
2. a
3. n
4. g
5. k
6. m
7. f
8. i
9. l
10. b
11. d
12. h
13. e
14. o
15. c

EXERCISE 2: LINKING IDEAS
1. elements
2. target population
3. sample, accessible population, and target population
4. You might identify any of the following:
   a. Compare the demographic characteristics of the sample with those of the target population determined from previous research.
   b. Compare mean sample values of study variables with the values of the target population determined from previous research.
   c. Identify the refusal rate in a study and the reasons potential study participants refused to be in the study. The lower the refusal rate and the more common the reasons for refusing to participate, the more representative the sample is of the target population.
   d. Evaluate the possibilities of systematic bias in the sample in terms of the setting, characteristics of the sample, and ranges of values on measured variables.
   e. Determine sample attrition rate and identify the reasons for the attrition or withdrawal of participants from the study. The lower the attrition rate and the more common or usual the reasons for attrition, the more representative the sample is of the target population.
5. Strength because random variation in participants' scores is important to accurately reflect the relationships among variables and limit the potential for error.

6. sampling frame
7. strategies or method(s) used to obtain a sample for a study
8. You might choose any of the following:
   a. Was the sampling plan adequately identified?
   b. Did the researcher successfully implement the sampling plan?
   c. Was the sampling plan effective in achieving representativeness of the target population?
   d. Were the participants selected from a sampling frame?
   e. Were the participants randomly selected?
9. homogeneous
10. heterogeneous
11. sampling criteria
12. sample characteristics
13. Sample attrition rate calculation: $(7 \div 65) \times 100\% = 0.1077 \times 100\% = 10.77\%$ or 10.8%.
    The sample attrition is a study strength because the rate is limited (approximately 11%).
    In addition, the reasons for attrition were common, which limits the potential impact on the study findings.
14. Types of random sampling
    a. simple random sampling
    b. stratified random sampling
    c. cluster sampling
    d. systematic sampling
15. You might list any of the following:
    a. convenience sampling
    b. network sampling
    c. purposive sampling
    d. theoretical sampling
16. nonprobability
17. power analysis
18. differences or relationships
19. 0.8 or 80%
20. null hypothesis
21. You might list any of the following:
    a. effect size of a study
    b. type of study
    c. study design
    d. number of variables
    e. measurement sensitivity
    f. data analysis techniques
22. You might list any of the following:
    a. data saturation
    b. scope of the study
    c. nature of the topic
    d. quality of the information collected
    e. study design

23. inclusion and exclusion
24. Refusal number = 250 − 208 = 42. Refusal rate = (42 refused ÷ 250 approached) × 100% = 0.168 × 100% = 16.8%
25. Attrition rate = (20 withdrew from the study ÷ 150 sample size) × 100% = 0.133 × 100% = 13.3%

Sampling Methods for Quantitative and Qualitative Studies

1. b
2. f
3. c
4. a
5. d
6. g
7. h
8. b
9. e
10. d and/or i
11. f
12. c
13. d
14. b
15. f
16. h
17. i
18. a
19. b
20. d and/or i

Determining Sample Size for Quantitative and Qualitative Studies

1. a
2. c
3. b
4. a
5. b
6. b
7. c
8. b
9. a
10. b

EXERCISE 3: WEB-BASED INFORMATION AND RESOURCES

1. You might have identified a variety of websites that discussed power analysis and provided a power analysis calculator. For example, G*Power provides an online program for understanding and conducting power analysis. Locate the free software at http://www.softpedia.com/get/Science-CAD/G-Power.shtml
   Some websites have useful information about research methodology; however, review the websites for quality. University websites usually provide more credible information than websites advertising products or services. Some websites will direct you to research articles and books that focus on power analysis and these could be excellent sources of information.
2. Your answer will depend on which website you selected. YouTube videos start with https://www.youtube.com/watch. Compare your answers with those of your peers to identify helpful video.

3. Yes, the content was similar to Grove and Gray (2023) textbook. For example, the URL https://www.youtube.com/watch?v=mlcdiVyVRSc discussed the snowball, purposive, and convenience sampling methods used in qualitative research.
4. Website for the GEOPoll Blog is https://www.geopoll.com/blog/probability-and-non-probability-samples/
5. The probability samples compared in the blog entry was the simple random sample and stratified random sample.
6. Website provided by World Health Organization (WHO) that provides quick links to COVID-19 information is: https://www.who.int/emergencies/diseases/novel-coronavirus-2019
7. Healthy People 2030 Objects and Data website is https://health.gov/healthypeople/objectives-and-data
8. Website for the National Center for Health Statistics: https://www.cdc.gov/nchs/index.htm
9. Centers for Disease Control and Prevention hosts the National Center for Health Statistics

EXERCISE 4: CONDUCTING CRITICAL APPRAISALS TO BUILD AN EVIDENCE-BASED PRACTICE

Steffen et al. (2021) Study

1. The study population included individuals with Type 2 diabetes mellitus (T2DM) and an associated diagnosis of arterial hypertension (AH).
2. "The inclusion criteria were being aged ≥ 18 years, having a medical diagnosis of T2DM associated with AH, and being registered in the programmatic actions of the study units in Risk Strata 3 and 4. The exclusion criteria were refusal to sign the informed consent form, patient not found after 3 attempts to contact by phone or in person at home, and illiteracy or a medical diagnosis of mental and behavioral disorders with impaired mental faculties" (Steffen et al., 2021, p. e204).
3. Yes, the sampling criteria were clearly stated and appropriate to designate the target population and to address the purpose of this study. Participants were included if they met the inclusion criteria and did not have the exclusion criteria.
4. Recruitment of study participants: "Recruiters were trained community health agents who used a single, standardized invitation model that followed the process of scheduling appointments, without any differentiation between the groups" (Steffen et al., 2021, p. e204).

5. Nonprobability sampling. Note that this randomized controlled trial (RCT) refers to the random assignment of participants into intervention and usual care groups (see Figure 1) and not random sampling to obtain participants.
6. Convenience sampling was used because participants in the selected health units who were willing to participate in the study were included in the sample.
7. The sociodemographic and health history characteristics for the participants in this study were presented in Table 1 (see pp. e207-e208). You may have listed any of the following characteristics: sex, age, race/ethnicity, living status (lives alone), educational level, marital status, per capita income, AH diagnosis time, T2DM diagnosis time, CVD family history, associated diseases, polypharmacy, depression symptoms, smoking, alcohol consumption, and time of physical exercise per week.
8. Yes, the sample was representative of the target population. The groups were similar, not significantly different, for the sample characteristic except for the nurse consultation that was managed during data analysis. A nonrandom sampling method was conducted in the study that reduced the sample's representativeness. However, the use of different health units that were selected based on their similarity increased the representativeness of the sample. Sample attrition was less than 10% for the total sample and groups increasing the representativeness. Therefore, the sample seemed representative of the target population in this study.
9. A sample of 189 participants stared the study and 174 participants completed the study.
10. Attrition rate for the sample = (15 withdrew from the study ÷ 189 sample size) × 100% = 0.079 × 100% = 7.9% rounded to 8%. Attrition rate for the usual care group = (8 withdrew from the usual care group ÷ 88 group size) × 100% = 0.0909 × 100% = 9.1% rounded to 9%. Attrition for the Test/MI group = (7 withdrew from the Test/MI group ÷ 101 group size) × 100% = 0.0693 × 100% = 6.9% rounded to 7%.
11. Yes, a rationale was provided for attrition in Figure 1, which included change in address, death, not found, and refusal. These reasons for lost to follow-up were basically the same for both groups, except the one participant who refused to continue in the usual care group. Steffen et al. (2021, p. e206 & e208) reported: "Losses to follow-up were balanced between the

groups and were attributed to death, refusal, or delay in collecting the outcomes within the period stipulated for completion of the study and change of address/inability to locate the subject, making it impossible to collect the final data (Figure 1). The measurement of the main outcome involved blood tests, and blood samples had to be collected in another outpatient clinic, so these were factors that led to dropout." Yes, the discussion of attrition was a strength, which was similar for the usual care group (9%) and the Test/MI group (7%). In addition, the reasons for attrition were common and similar for both groups.

12. No the sample size was not adequate for the Steffen et al. (2021) study. The initial sample was 189. A power analysis was conducted prior to data collection to determine what would be an adequate sample size. "Because of the absence of a pilot study, a study with a similar research protocol was used to anticipate the expected effect size. On the basis of that study, investigators added 10% for possible losses and refusals, and the sample size was estimated at 248 patients by Winpepi, version 11.61. The authors considered a power of 80%, a significance level of 5%, and an *SD* of 2% for a mean difference of 0.75% in HbA1c" (Steffen et al., 2021, p. e204). The researchers acknowledged in the Limitation section that the ideal sample size was not reached because of limited study resources. They reported this smaller sample might have resulted in an altered estimation of population parameters and reduced effect of the intervention. In addition, the groups were not significantly different for the dependent variable HbA1c, which might be a Type II error from an inadequate sample size.

13. No, the study findings are not ready to generalize to the target population or to use in practice. Steffen et al., 2021, p. e211) reported: "Nevertheless, additional evidence is needed to examine and support the forms of implementation of MI in primary care with larger and more representative samples for evaluating the effects on the professional skills and on the knowledge, attitudes, and outcomes of patients with T2DM, particularly in HbA1c levels." The generalizability of the study findings is limited by the nonprobability sampling method used, and the HbA1c levels were not significantly different between the groups.

14. Study setting: The setting was clearly identified as health units in Brazil and would be considered a partially controlled setting. "The health units were selected on the basis of the similarity of epidemiologic profile and health indicators in T2DM and AH" (Steffen et al., 2021, p. e204).

15. Yes, the setting was appropriate for this RCT, because the similar, large health units were selected to ensure a large, homogenous sample to examine the effect of the intervention.

Colwill et al. (2021) Study

1. The population was identified in the study title as "patients with intravenous drug use/abuse-related endocarditis" (Colwill et al., 2021).

2. Sampling criteria: "Inclusion criteria were adult PWID [persons who inject drugs] hospitalized with endocarditis undergoing evaluation for surgical management. Those who could not participate in an in-person interview conducted in English were excluded" (Colwill et al., 2021, Participants section). The sampling criteria were appropriate for recruiting participants to address the research question and aim identified in the study (see Study Guide Chapter 5 critical appraisal).

3. Recruitment of participants: "Potential participants were identified from patient lists of those undergoing surgical evaluation for endocarditis. The electronic medical record was reviewed to identify those with a diagnosis of substance use/abuse disorder and individuals were approached for participation" (Colwill et al., 2021, Procedures section).

4. nonprobability sampling

5. Colwill et al. (2021, Participants section) reported that "theoretical purposive sampling methods were used."

6. The sample characteristics for this study were presented in Table 1. In addition, Colwill et al. (2021, Results section) reported: "Eleven participants… were interviewed over a period of one year. The sample was female (5), Caucasian (7), married (3), and employed (3)." The demographic variables were (gender, age, marital status, education, race, employment, household income, and place of residence).

7. You might have answered yes or no. Yes, the demographic variables seemed appropriate to describe the sample. However, only eight of the participants provided the majority of the demographic information. Three participants did not report most of their demographic information. The sample characteristics were adequate but limited for some of the participants.

8. Sample size was $n = 11$ PWID

9. Yes, the sample size of 11 was adequate for this grounded theory study. The sample size is within a range typical for a qualitative study; and more importantly, the sample size was based on data saturation. Colwill et al. (2021, Data analysis section) reported: "Theoretical saturation was reached when, concepts of the emerging model with no new themes surfaced and, the team developed a good understanding of the recurring themes (Sbaraini et al., 2011). Discrepancies were resolved through iterations, numerous discussions, and going back to the data."

10. Setting: "This study was conducted in the inpatient setting within a quaternary care medical center in the Midwest" (Colwill et al., 2021, Participants section). Yes, this setting was appropriate because 11 of the patients in this hospital met the sampling criteria and were included in this study. These participants provided quality information to address the study research question and aim. In addition, private, convenient patient rooms were provided for conducting the study interviews.

Greene and Ramos (2021) Study

1. The population was patients of usual healthcare providers.

2. The quantitative part of the Greene and Ramos (2021) study was a secondary data analysis and sometimes the sampling criteria used for the primary data collection are not presented. However, the study would be strengthened by a more detailed discussion of the original study and the data collected. The researchers did indicate they selected from the total database of $>9,000$ persons who had a usual healthcare provider and had provided data on the key study variables.

3. The sample characteristics for the Greene and Ramos (2021) study are presented in Table 1, which provided description of the demographic variables gender, age, education, income, race/ethnicity, and health insurance for both the quantitative and qualitative parts of the study.

4. Yes, the researchers did provide a clear description of the participants for both the interview and survey participants. "Qualitative interview participants were disproportionately Black, lower income, and female (Table 1). Almost half (48%) had incomes at or below 138% of the federal poverty level (FPL), and only a quarter had incomes at or above 250% FPL" (Greene & Ramos, 2021, p. 1224). Thus, the use of purposive sampling was affective in obtaining the distribution of participates desired for the qualitative part of this study.

5. Nonprobability sampling method was used for the quantitative part of the Greene and Ramos (2021) study. The participants' with usual healthcare providers and no missing data for key variables were included from the HRMS database. This method is consistent with convenience sampling.

6. Yes, the sample size for the quantitative part of the study was adequate, $n = 6,392$ (see Table 1). This was a secondary data analysis so a very large sample size was achieved. Greene and Ramos (2021, p. 1224) clarified the sample size in the following quote: "Of the 9,811 survey respondents, 6,666 (69%) had a usual health care provider. Our sample of 6,392 excluded those with missing data on key variables." The sample for the quantitative part of this study was extremely strong and provided significant findings. All correlation values had a p-value <0.01, so no evidence of a type II error was noted (see Table 2).

7. The inclusion criteria for the qualitative part of this study are best represented by the following statement: "Participants were respondents to the March 2018 HRMS [Health Reform Monitoring Survey], who had a usual health care provider and indicated on the survey a willingness to participate in a follow up telephone interview" (Greene & Ramos, 2021, p. 1223).

8. No, the sampling criteria for the qualitative part of this study were not clearly labeled or identified. The inclusion sampling criteria in this study were limited as indicated in the answer to Question 7. No exclusion sampling criteria were noted.

9. Nonprobability sampling method was used in the qualitative part of this study. Greene and Ramos (2021, p. 1223) reported: "We oversampled Black respondents and those with lower incomes ($< = 138\%$ federal poverty level) because of evidence that those groups have lower trust in health providers. We additionally oversampled those reporting low trust in their usual provider in the HRMS." This quote indicates that purposeful or purposive sampling was used in this study but no specific sampling method was identified.

10. Sample size for the qualitative part of the study was $n = 40$. A sample size of 40 participants is considered strong for most

qualitative studies (Grove & Gray, 2023). In addition, the data collected was adequate to address the study purpose focused on "identifying the key health care provider behaviors that patients reported build their trust, as well as those that lose their trust" (Greene & Ramons, 2021, p. 1223).

11. Greene and Ramos (2021, p. 1223) reported that they "conducted 40 semi-structured telephone interviews." The setting would be considered nature because the telephone interviews were conducted at a site chosen by the participant, probably their homes.

CHAPTER 10—CLARIFYING MEASUREMENT AND DATA COLLECTION IN QUANTITATIVE RESEARCH

EXERCISE 1: TERMS AND DEFINITIONS

Measurement Concepts and Methods

1.	g	9.	d
2.	o	10.	a
3.	h	11.	e
4.	n	12.	c
5.	l	13.	f
6.	j	14.	b
7.	m	15.	i
8.	k		

Reliability, Validity, Accuracy, and Precision in Measurement

1.	l	8.	h
2.	a	9.	c
3.	n	10.	i
4.	e	11.	f
5.	m	12.	k
6.	g	13.	b
7.	d	14.	j

Data Collection

1.	c	4.	a
2.	b	5.	e
3.	d		

EXERCISE 2: LINKING IDEAS

1. ratio-level of measurement
2. 0.8
3. ordinal (The stages of breast cancer can be rank ordered according to level of severity.)
4. unequal; equal

5. a self-report form designed to elicit information through written, verbal, or electronic responses from study participants.
6. Cronbach alpha
7. reliable; New scales with a Cronbach alpha of 0.70 are considered reliable (Grove & Cipher, 2020; Grove & Gray, 2023). As a scale is used in additional studies, the reliability will be examined and items will be revised as needed to improve the reliability and validity of the scale.
8. reliability and validity
9. it is not valid
10. interval
11. unstructured
12. structured
13. Personal interview because they have close to a 100% response rate and mailed questionnaires usually have a low response rate, approximately 30-40% (Waltz et al., 2017).
14. predictive validity and concurrent validity
15. You might have listed any of the following or might have another idea that results in measurement error.
    a. Scale or questionnaire items lack reliability.
    b. Poorly developed scale or questionnaire that lacks validity.
    c. Scale lacks reliability or validity testing in the study population.
    d. Physiological measure that lacks precision in the measurement of a study variable.
    e. Physiological measure that lacks accuracy in the measurement of a study variable.
    f. Physiological equipment is not maintained or recalibrated as recommended by the manufacturer.
    g. Study participants are unable to read and understand the items on a scale because the reading level is too high or complex for them.
    h. Variations in administration of the measurement method. For example, the person taking the measurements may not use the same procedure every time.
    i. Study participants leaving an item blank accidentally on a measurement scale.
    j. Participant completing a scale on a computer accidentally hits the wrong key when entering an answer.
    k. Participants misreading or misunderstanding an item on a measurement method.
    l. Hitting the wrong key when entering data into the computer.
    m. Disorganization during data entry into a computer.

Measurement Error

1. b   4. b
2. a   5. a
3. a

Levels of Measurement

1. c   11. d
2. a   12. a
3. d   13. b
4. b or c (degree or   14. d
   years of education)   15. a
5. a   16. b
6. b   17. d
7. d   18. b
8. d   19. a
9. c   20. a
10. a

Scales

1. a
2. c
3. b

Sensitivity and Specificity

Completion of the table on sensitivity and specificity.

Diagnostic Test Results	Disease Present	Disease Absent or Not Present
Positive test	a (true positive)	b (false positive)
Negative test	c (false negative)	d (true negative)

1. Formula for sensitivity: $a/(a + c)$ = True positive rate
2. Formula for specificity: $d/(b + d)$ = True negative rate
3. 50
4. $(50 \div 300) \times 100\% = 0.166 \times 100\% = 16.667\% = 16.67\%$
5. 40
6. $(40 \div 790) \times 100\% = 0.0506 \times 100\% = 5.06\%$
7. Sensitivity = $250/(250 + 40) \times 100\% = 250/290 \times 100\% = 0.86206 \times 100 = 86.21\%$
8. The sensitivity value is strong at 86.21% in identifying a patient with the disease.
9. Specificity = $750/(50 + 750) \times 100\% = 750/800 \times 100\% = 0.9375 \times 100\% = 93.75\%$
10. Positive LR = sensitivity ÷ (100% – specificity)
11. Positive LR = $86.2\% \div (100\% – 93.75\%) = 86.2\% \div 6.25\% = 13.792\% = 13.79\%$
12. The positive LR of 13.79% is strong to rule in a disease because it is > 10, which indicates that the patient has the disease when the test is positive.
13. Negative LR = (100% – sensitivity) ÷ specificity
14. Negative LR = $(100\% – 86.2\%) \div 93.75\% = 13.8\% \div 93.75\% = 0.147 = 0.15$
15. The negative LR of 0.15 is fairly strong to rule out a disease because it is close to the value of < 0.1 that indicates the likelihood that the patient does not have the disease when the test is negative.

EXERCISE 3: WEB-BASED INFORMATION AND RESOURCES

1. https://www.ahrq.gov/evidencenow/index.html
2. EvidenceNow projects are an AHRQ solution for revitalizing the Nation's primary care system.
3. https://www.ahrq.gov/priority-populations/index.html
4. The priority populations identified by AHRQ included: Children/adolescents, elderly, low-income, rural/inner-city residents, special healthcare needs, and women.
5. You might have identified one of the following websites or others that discuss the CES-R: http://cesd-r.com/; http://cesd-r.com/cesdr/
6. You might have identified one of the following websites or another one: https://www.brightfutures.org/mentalhealth/pdf/professionals/bridges/ces_dc.pdf http://www.ncbi.nlm.nih.gov/pubmed/2301363
7. http://www.wongbakerfaces.org/
8. Whelton, P. K., Carey, R. M., Aronow, W. S., Casey, D. E., Collins, K. J., Himmelfarb, C. D. ... Wright, J. W. (2018). 2017 Guideline for the Prevention, Detection, Evaluation, and Management of High Blood Pressure in Adults: Executive summary: A report of the American College of Cardiology/American Heart Association task force on clinical practice guidelines. *Hypertension, 71*(6), 1269-1324. https://doi.org/10.1161/HYP.0000000000000066
9. http://hrms.urban.org/
10. "The Health Reform Monitoring Survey (HRMS) is a survey of the nonelderly population that is exploring the value of cutting-edge Internet-based survey methods to monitor the Affordable Care Act (ACA) before data from federal government surveys are available. Funding for the core HRMS is provided by the Robert Wood Johnson Foundation and the Urban Institute" (see http://hrms.urban.org/) website.

EXERCISE 4: CONDUCTING CRITICAL APPRAISALS TO BUILD AN EVIDENCE-BASED PRACTICE

Steffen et al. (2021) Study

1. Steffen et al. (2021) study variables, measurement methods, and directness of measurement.

Variables	Measurement Methods	Direct or Indirect Measurement Method
Hemoglobin A1c (HbA1c))	Laboratory test of blood sample	Direct
*Systolic blood pressure (SBP)	BP equipment in the Health Unit	Direct
*Diastolic blood pressure (DBP)	BP equipment in the Health Unit	Direct

* You might have listed only blood pressure (BP), which is acceptable but the analysis was conduct on both systolic and diastolic BPs.

2. "HbA1c was measured through laboratory tests of blood samples collected in the outpatient department, following the routine practices of these services and without any differentiation between the groups" (Steffen et al., 2021, p. e206).

3. Critical appraisal HbA1c measurements: Steffen et al. (2021) reported the blood samples were collected in a routine way for both groups in the outpatient department, which supported the precision and accuracy of the HbA1c values. However, the researchers needed to expand on who collected the blood samples and how. Interrater reliability of the data collectors needed to be calculated to ensure consistent data collection. In addition, there was no discussion of how the blood samples were transferred from the outpatient department to the lab. The accuracy of the laboratory equipment in analyzing blood samples and reporting values needed to be addressed. Did the lab meet national standards, was it certified? The accuracy and potential for errors in determining the HbA1c values within the lab also needed to be discussed. Limited information was provided regarding the accuracy and precision of the HbA1c values in this study. The researchers need to consider if the quality of the HbA1c

measurements might have contributed to the nonsignificant outcomes for the HbA1c in this study.

4. "Blood pressure (BP) [was] measured in the Health Unit by nursing technicians who were not included in the study team; following the routine and technical guidelines inherent to the procedure, without differentiation between the groups" (Steffen et al., 2021, p. e206).

5. Critical appraisal of BP measurements: The discussion of the process for measuring participants' BPs lacked acceptable detail. The training of the nurse technicians on BP measurement was not described. In addition, the interrater reliability of these technicians for taking and reporting BP values should be detailed to support the precision of the measurement process. Steffen et al. (2021) reported technical guidelines were followed for taking BPs, but were these the most current international guidelines for measuring BPs described by Whelton et al. (2018). This source was presented earlier in the Web-Based Information section. The equipment for taking BPs was not described so the accuracy could not be determined. Thus, the researchers provided very limited information about the precision and accuracy of the BP measurements.

6. Extraneous or confounding variables

Extraneous or Confounding Variable	Name of the Measurement Method	Type of Measurement Method
Depression	Beck Depression Inventory	Likert scale
Adherence	Martin-Bayarre-Grade Questionnaire	Likert Scale

7. Rationale for measuring cofounding variables: "Because of the correlation among adherence, motivation, and depression in chronic diseases, symptoms of depression were measured at baseline as a risk factor for poorer clinical outcomes and therefore were a possible confounder" (Steffen et al., 2021, p. e206). Depression and adherence, considered confounding or extraneous variables, were measured to determine their influence on the outcome variables, HbA1c and BP.

8. Critical appraisal Beck Depression Inventory (BDI): "The Beck Depression Inventory is a self-report and depression screening instrument composed of 21 items, including symptoms and attitudes, in which 20 points is the cut off differentiating a higher level of depressive symptoms (Steffen et al., 2021, p. e206). No reliability information is provided for the BDI from previous research or for this current study. Only criterion-related validity of the concurrent type is provided from previous research that determined the 20 point cut off for higher levels of depressive symptoms (Grove & Gray, 2023). Thus, the BDI can be administer to adults in clinical settings and determine those with probable depression. The discussion of the reliability and validity of the BDI is inadequate in this study for you to critically appraise.

9. Data collection process: "Study participants were individuals with T2DM and an associated diagnosis of AH, were registered in the health units established as the research settings… Simple individual randomization was performed electronically by… a professional who was not part of the study team. The professional randomized and allocated all possible eligible patients into 2 groups—test/MI group and usual-care group—before the research team initiated recruitment. Participants allocated in each group were recruited in ascending order, and if they met the inclusion criteria… Recruiters were trained community health agents who used a single, standardized invitation model that followed the process of scheduling appointments, without any differentiation between the groups. On acceptance to participate, individuals received at home a brown envelope with the informed consent form and instructions for the start of interventions from the community health agent" (Steffen et al., 2021, p. e204).

"Before and after the training, nurses filled out 3 validated questionnaires to assess the importance and confidence in the use of MI and their mastery of the initial basic skills to apply MI in practice… The outcomes were measured at baseline and at 3 months after the second nursing consultation as final outcomes. The measurements were conducted in a blinded form, except for the participant profile questionnaire, which was completed by a nurse during the interventions because it contained important clinical data that required confirmation and updating of these records in the patient's medical records" (Steffen et al., 2021, p. e206).

10. Critical appraisal of data collection process: Steffen et al (2021) provided extensive detail regarding the recruitment and selection of study participants. The process for assigning participants to groups was detailed as was the process for training nurses for implementing the Test/MI intervention. The researchers needed to provide more information about the measurement methods and the process for collecting data from the study participants.

Greene and Ramos (2021) Study

1. "We conducted secondary analysis of the Health Reform Monitoring Survey (HRMS) to examine the relationship between trust and the key components of trust identified in the qualitative component" (Greene & Ramos, 2021, p. 1223).

2. Data for this study were obtained from HRMS that was a national survey conducted in the United States with a 62% response rate. The sample equaled 6,392 participants for the quantitative part of this study and included only surveys that were complete on the key variables. Greene and Ramos (2021) do not provide specific information about the development of the HRMS, nor do they provide reliability and validity information for this survey. This is common when doing a secondary analysis of data. Having located the website for the HRMS in the previous section, you know this survey was developed for adults to monitor the outcomes of the Affordable Care Act and was funded by the Robert Wood Johnson Foundation and the Urban Institute. This information adds to the credibility of the survey data. However, the researchers needed to strengthen the measurement section by providing more information about the HRMS.

3. When conducing a secondary data analysis, researchers need to review the measurement method used to collect the original data. The

data must be examined to ensure that the research purpose and objectives or questions are addressed by the data. The data needs to be complete for the variables studied, which was ensured by Greene and Ramos (2021).

4. "Trust was measured by asking respondents how much they agreed or disagreed with the following statement: "I trust my doctor (provider)" using a 5 point agree-disagree scale" (Greene & Ramos, 2021, p. 1224). Examining trust with a 5 point scale of agree-disagree is typical of a Likert scale but most Likert scales have 10-20 items to measure a concept. The researchers do not identify the type of scale used to measure trust in this study.

5. The quantitative part of the Greene and Ramos (2021) study was a secondary data analysis so quantitative data were not collected in this study. The data collection process focused on the 40 semi-structured interviews that were conducted during the qualitative part of this study (see Study Guide Chapters 3 and 14).

CHAPTER 11—UNDERSTANDING STATISTICS IN RESEARCH

EXERCISE 1: TERMS AND DEFINITIONS

1.	e	9.	b
2.	c	10.	f
3.	o	11.	g
4.	d	12.	k
5.	a	13.	l
6.	m	14.	h
7.	i	15.	j
8.	n		

EXERCISE 2: LINKING IDEAS

1. Statistical analyses are techniques or procedures conducted to examine, consolidate, and give meaning to the numerical data gathered in a study.
2. You might have listed any three of the following:
   a. manage missing data
   b. describe the sample and study variables
   c. examine reliability of measurement methods
   d. conduct exploratory data analysis to identify outliers
   e. examine the distribution of data in a study for normality
   f. conduct inferential statistical analysis
   g. conduct post hoc analyses if required

3. You might have listed any three of the following analysis techniques:
   a. Estimates of central tendency, such as mode, median, and mean
   b. Estimates of dispersion, such as range, variance, and standard deviation
   c. Examination of data to identify outliers
   d. Frequencies and percentages are calculated for nominal and ordinal data to determine the occurrence of demographic variables. For example, with a sample size of 250, the sample was 128 (51.2%) female and 122 (48.8%) male.
   e. Differences among groups are examined to demonstrate equivalence at the start of the study.

4. Results from statistical analyses in quasi-experimental and experimental studies.
   a. significant and predicted results
   b. nonsignificant results
   c. significant and unpredicted results
   d. mixed results
   e. unexpected results

5. You might have listed any of the following:
   a. findings
   b. comparison of the findings from the current study to the findings from previous studies
   c. limitations
   d. conclusions
   e. generalization of findings
   f. implications for nursing
   g. recommendations for further study

6. The normal curve is a symmetrical curve where the mean, median, and mode fall at the same point. Figure 11-1 in Chapter 11 of your textbook, *Understanding Nursing Research*, 8th edition, includes a drawing of the normal curve with a mean of 0 and a standard deviation of 1.

7. 95%
8. one-tailed test of significance
9. Type I error
10. group differences
11. mode
12. standard deviation
13. the group size
14. scatterplot
15. bivariate analysis

Linking Statistics With Analysis Techniques

1.	c	6.	i
2.	f	7.	h
3.	g	8.	e
4.	a	9.	b
5.	d	10.	j

Linking Levels of Measurement With Analysis Techniques

1. c
2. a
3. c
4. c
5. a and b
6. b
7. c
8. c
9. c
10. b and c
11. a
12. a and b
13. c
14. c
15. b

Statements, Inferences, and Generalizations

1. d
2. b
3. a
4. c

Describing the Sample

1. Age in years
2. Bachelor of Science in Nursing (BSN)
3. 40–49 years
4. Standard deviation (SD) = 2.1
5. 35 years of experience that is identified in the range
6. 95% = Mean $\pm$ 1.96(SD) = 15.5 $\pm$ 1.96(2.1) = 15.5 $\pm$ 4.12 = (11.38, 19.62)

Measures of Central Tendency

1. 3.42
2. 3.10
3. 3.00 because this score is the most frequent value (mode) in this distribution of scores.
4. Mean $\pm$ SD = 3.42 + 0.76 = 4.18 and 3.42 – 0.76 = 2.66
   2.66 to 4.18 or (2.66, 4.18)

Name That Statistical Analysis Technique!

1. d—Analysis of variance (ANOVA) is conducted to determine group differences for three or more groups, interval or ratio level data
2. a—Chi-square analysis is conducted to determine whether two variables are independent or related in a study, nominal level data
3. c—Pearson correlation is conducted to examine relationships between variables in a study, interval or ratio level data
4. b—t-test is conducted to determine a difference between two groups in a study, interval or ratio level data

Significance of Results

1. NS
2. *
3. *
4. NS
5. *

EXERCISE 3: WEB-BASED INFORMATION AND RESOURCES

1. The following websites address power analysis calculation and you might have identified other sites for power analysis:
   a. http://power-analysis.com/ *Power and Precision* provides free software to calculate power analysis.
   b. http://powerandsamplesize.com/ *Free, Online, Easy-to-Use Power and Sample Size Calculators*
   c. *Sample size calculator:* https://www.surveymonkey.com/mp/sample-size-calculator/
2. *Making sense of statistical power*: https://www.americannursetoday.com/making-sense-of-statistical-power/
3. SPSS stands for Statistical Package for the Social Sciences
4. You might have identified one of the following websites or another that addresses introduction to SPSS:
   a. SPSS software: www.ibm/com/softwre/analytics/spss/
   b. Social Science Computing Cooperative (SSCC): http://ssc.wisc.edu/sscc/pubs/spss/classintro/spss_students1.html
   c. How to analyze data using SPSS: https://www.wikihow.com/Analyse-Data-Using-SPSS
   d. Introduction to SPSS on YouTube: https://www.youtube.com/watch?v=msI7xf0tInE
5. Amazon website for the Grove and Cipher (2020) text:
   Statistics for Nursing Research: A Workbook for Evidence-Based Practice: 9780323654111: Medicine & Health Science Books @ Amazon.com
6. https://www.sas.com/en_us/home.html
7. Number Cruncher Statistical System (NCSS): www.ncss.com

EXERCISE 4: CONDUCTING CRITICAL APPRAISALS TO BUILD AN EVIDENCE-BASED PRACTICE

Steffen et al. (2021) Study

1. The study included two groups: the test/MI group (treatment or intervention group) and the usual-care group (comparison group).
2. Study participants were randomly assigned to the test/MI and usual-care groups. The "randomization was performed electronically by the SSC/GHC Monitoring Evaluation center by a professional who was not part of the study team" (Steffen et al., 2021, p. e204).

3. The groups were independent. Randomizing participants into groups results in independent groups, because the assignment of individuals to one group or another is unrelated (Grove & Gray, 2023).

4. Link of variables, level of measurement, and descriptive data analysis techniques:

Demographic Variables	Level of Measurement	Descriptive Analysis Techniques
Sex (Gender)	Nominal	Frequency, percentage
Age	Ratio	Mean, standard deviation
Race/ethnicity	Nominal	Frequency, percentage
Lives alone, yes	Nominal	Frequency, percentage
Educational level	Nominal	Frequency, percentage
Marital status	Nominal	Frequency, percentage
Cardiovascular disease family history, yes	Nominal	Frequency, percentage
Depression symptoms by the Beck Depression Inventory (BDI), positive score*	Nominal	Frequency, percentage
Smoking	Nominal	Frequency, percentage
Consultation with a nurse in the previous year (yes or no)	Nominal	Frequency, percentage

* Multi-item scales such as the BDI are considered to have interval level data but in this study the data were nominal with the focus on identifying those participants who were depressed (had a positive score). The variable was depressed/not depressed (nominal categories).

5. a. Yes, one characteristic was significantly different between the two groups, "consultation with a nurse in the previous year" ($p = 0.02$) (Steffen et al., 2021, p. e208). All other demographic characteristics were not significantly different between the two groups with p-values > 0.05 (Table 1; Steffen et al., 2021, pp. e207-e208).

    b. The groups being similar at the start of the study is a strength. The sample characteristics that are not significantly different between the two groups indicate the groups were similar for these characteristics at the start of the study. Any effect of the demographic variables on the outcome variables will be similar between the groups. Thus, any significant changes at the completion of the study are more likely to be caused by the study treatment or intervention rather than original group differences (Grove & Cipher, 2020).

    c. Steffen et al. (2021, p. e208) reported: "consultation with the nurse in the previous year, which was statistically adjusted as described in the data analysis because it represented a higher amount of intervention received by the usual-care group from baseline." This is a study weakness that was managed statistically to reduce the effect on the study findings.

6. Description of study outcome variables in the following table.

Outcome or Dependent Variables	Level of Measurement	Descriptive Analysis Techniques
Hemoglobin A1c (HbA1c)	Ratio	Mean, standard deviation
Systolic blood pressure (SBP)	Ratio	Mean, standard deviation
Diastolic blood pressure (DBP)	Ratio	Mean, standard deviation

7. The inferential statistic conducted to examine group differences was the t-test. This analysis technique was appropriate because the variables were ratio level measurement and the focus was examining differences between two groups for the HbA1c, SBP, and DBP outcomes.

8. There was no statistically significant difference in the HbA1c levels ($p = 0.07$) between the groups. The Test/MI intervention did not show a significant improvement in HbA1c levels between the experiment and usual care groups. The researchers reported that the study limitations might have affected these results and additional research is needed to test the effectiveness of the intervention on HbA1c.

9. Steffen et al. (2021, p. e210) provided the following rationale for the nonsignificant HbA1c results between the two groups: "Better

outcomes could be achieved by professionals with higher levels of training and experience. … Furthermore, the ideal sample size was not reached because of the lack of resources for the research. … The inclusion of all participants regardless of whether their baseline HbA1c levels were within the therapeutic target, contributed to the prediction of the restricted margin for reduction, considering the baseline profile of the study population."

10. The SBP and DBP were significantly different between the Test/MI and usual-care groups at $p = 0.01$ for both variables (see Table 2; Steffen et al., 2021, p. e209). These results indicates that the Test/MI intervention was significantly effective in lowering the SBP and the DBP of the intervention group as compared to the usual-care group.

11. The HbA1c result in the Test/MI group
    a. Yes, the 0.4% reduction in the HbA1c for the Test/MI group from baseline to the end of the study was statistically significant because $p < 0.01$, which was smaller than the level of significance (alpha) that was set at 0.05 prior to the study.
    b. Yes, this result is clinically important because the HbA1c value improved for the intervention group almost a half of a percent. However, additional research is needed with correction of the study limitations to determine if the HbA1c levels would be statistically significant between the intervention and usual care groups.

12. Yes, the results were similar as reported by Steffen et al., 2021, p. e210): "Similar results were shown in studies that investigated MI in primary care environments on the basis of different modalities of delivery and with weak quality of evidence."

13. Steffen et al. (2021) detailed the limitations of their study on page e210 that focused on: Inadequate training experience for nurses delivering the intervention, inadequate sample size based on the power analysis results, participants included with HbA1c levels in therapeutic range, and complexity of people with chronic disease in primary care environment. As discussed earlier in Question 9, these limitations do help explain the study results regarding HbA1c.

14. Steffen et al. (2021) stressed the significant improvement in SBP and DBP in the intervention group making MI a useful

intervention in practice. However, due to the nonsignificant results between the groups for the HbA1c levels, addition research should be conducted focusing on reducing the study limitations. Thus, either answers of using the intervention in practice now or recommending additional research before use in practice are acceptable.

15. Some the suggestions for further research by Steffen et al. (2021, p. e211) included: "Additional evidence is needed to examine and support the forms of implementation of MI in primary care with larger and more representative samples for evaluating the effects on the professional skills and on the knowledge, attitudes, and outcomes of patients with T2DM, particularly in HbA1c levels…. Finally, qualitative scientific methodologies should be included to determine how people receiving treatment for hypertension and diabetes who receive MI and the professionals who apply MI feel about it." Yes, these suggestions are appropriate based on the study findings and limitations.

Greene and Ramos (2021) Study

1. Link of variables, level of measurement, and descriptive analysis techniques (Table 1; Greene & Ramos, 2021, p. 1223).

Demographic Variables	Level of Measurement	Descriptive Analysis Techniques
Gender	Nominal	Frequency, percentage
Age (ranges)	Ordinal	Frequency, percentage
Income (% of federal poverty level)	Ordinal	Frequency, percentage
Race/ethnicity	Nominal	Frequency, percentage
Health insurance	Nominal	Frequency, percentage

2. Descriptive correlational design
3. Correlational analysis was conducted using the Spearman rank-order technique, which is conducted to analyze data at the ordinal level for relationships. Greene and Ramos (2021, p, 1222) reported: "We then analyzed a nationally representative survey ($n = 6,517$) to

examine the relationship between respondents' trust in their usual provider and the key trust-related behaviors identified in the qualitative interviews."

4. Relationship of trust in provider with one of the trust-related behaviors
   a. Yes, this relationship is significant because all the correlation values in Table 2 have *p*-values <0.01, which is below the level of significance of 0.05 set for the study (see the note at the bottom of Table 2).
   b. The correlational value of 0.69 represents a strong relationship (Grove & Gray, 2023).
   c. The correlational value is positive because there is no negative sign in front of the value. This positive correlational value means that the two concepts change together, one increases as the other increases or one decreases as the other decreases. Thus, as trust in one's provider increases, the belief the provider listens carefully to what I say increases.
   d. Explained variance is calculated by squaring the correlational value $(0.69)^2$ x 100% = 0.4761 x 100% = 47.6% or 48%

5. a. The lowest correlation is 0.52 between trust of provider and the behavior "my doctor/provider does not spend enough time with me" (Greene & Ramos, 2021, p. 1226). The scoring for this item was reversed.
   b. The correlation value 0.52 is a strong, positive relationship between trust in provider and provider spending enough time.

6. Limitations: Greene and Ramos (2021) study findings did not support the belief that people from racial/ethnic minority backgrounds and with lower incomes would report lower trust in their physician/provider. In this study, the trust in provider reported across race/ethnic minorities and income levels were consistent, not different. In addition, the researchers were unable to quantitatively test every element of their qualitive findings. The spending enough time with patients might have lowered the correlation with trust. This study only examined trust of their healthcare provider and not other issues related to trust such as trust in healthcare institutions, technology, and research.

7. Implications for practice: "Since trust is related to better patient health-related behaviors

and utilization, it is important for healthcare providers to actively listen, provide detailed explanations, show care and concern for patients and their health, and demonstrate their knowledge" (Greene & Ramos, 2021, p. 1227). These are appropriate implications for practice because these ideas are strongly supported by previous research. However the researchers also recognized these trust behaviors were sometimes challenging for providers to accomplish in current clinical practice.

8. Suggests for further research: "Future research should test whether strategies to improve health provider communication, like motivational interviewing, impact patient trust and health outcomes. Further, building trusting relationships with patients may not only have positive impacts on patients. Trusting patient-provider relationships may improve health care provider wellbeing, job fulfillment, as well as care team dynamics, and these relationships also warrant future investigation" (Greene & Ramos, 2021, p. 1227). Further research was also suggested to examine trust in healthcare institutions.

9. Conclusions: "Respondents in this study reported that trusting their health care provider was crucial for them to visit the provider, share personal information with the provider and follow through with the provider's advice. To earn their trust, participants said that health providers need to communicate effectively, express that they care about their patients and their patients' health, and demonstrate competence" (Greene & Ramos, 2021, p. 1227). Yes, these conclusions were appropriate because this study's findings were similar to the findings of previous research. In addition, a framework was developed as a basis for further research.

CHAPTER 12—CRITICAL APPRAISAL OF QUANTITATIVE AND QUALITATIVE RESEARCH FOR NURSING PRACTICE

EXERCISE 1: TERMS AND DEFINITIONS

1. i
2. h
3. b
4. g
5. j

6. d
7. c
8. a
9. e
10. f

EXERCISE 2: LINKING IDEAS

1. You might include any three of the following:
   a. What are the major strengths of the study?
   b. What are the major weaknesses of the study?
   c. Are the findings of the study an accurate reflection of reality?
   d. What is the significance of the findings for nursing practice?
   e. Are the findings consistent with those of previous studies?
2. You might list any of the following or have other ideas:
   a. Critically appraise studies for class assignments.
   b. Critically appraise research to share the findings with other healthcare professionals.
   c. Read and critically appraise studies to solve a problem in practice.
   d. Critically appraise studies in a selected area and summarize the findings for use in practice.
   e. Critically appraise a proposed study to determine whether it is ethical to conduct in your clinical agency.
3. rights, informed consent
4. Components of qualitative research abstract
   a. Purpose
   b. Qualitative approach
   c. Sample
   d. Key results

Determination of Quantitative Study Strengths and Weaknesses

1. W
2. S
3. W
4. W
5. S
6. W or S. Weakness (W) if the goal of sampling was to recruit a heterogeneous sample representing the target population. Network sampling could be a strength (S) if the sample was difficult to recruit because the topic was sexual abuse or other sensitive or stigmatized topics. In such cases, network sampling might be the only feasible strategy for recruiting an adequate number of participants.
7. S
8. S
9. W
10. S
11. W
12. S
13. W Only 48% of the studies were considered current (published in the last 10 years). Obesity is a severe health problem for many people and weight loss is the focus of many recent studies.
14. S
15. S

Determination of Qualitative Study Strengths and Weaknesses

1.	S	6.	S
2.	W	7.	S
3.	W	8.	S
4.	S	9.	S
5.	W	10.	W

11. S
12. W- Remember from Chapter 9 that exclusion criteria are not the opposite of each other. The exclusion criteria are reasons you would not allow a person to participate even though he or she met the inclusion criteria. In this example, the exclusion criteria could be persons who were taking more than two anti-hypertensive medications, had experienced a transient ischemic attack (TIA) in the past year, or had a history of a cerebrovascular accident (CVA).
13. S
14. W
15. S

EXERCISE 3: WEB-BASED INFORMATION AND RESOURCES

1. The QSEN website for pre-licensure nursing students is: http://qsen.org/competencies/pre-licensure-ksas/
2. Evidence-based practice (EBP) competency
3. EBP Attitude: "Appreciate strengths and weaknesses of scientific bases for practice" (QSEN, 2020). Retrieved from EBP section on the following website: http://qsen.org/competencies/pre-licensure-ksas/
4. EBP Skill: "Read original research and evidence reports related to area of practice" (QSEN, 2020).
5. CONSORT 20210 flow diagram for RCTs: http://www.consort-statement.org/consort-statement/flow-diagram
6. Critical Appraisal Skills Programme (CASP) website: https:casp-uk.net
7. CASP website for critical appraisal checklist for RCTs: https://casp-uk.b-cdn.net/wp-content/uploads/2020/10/CASP_RCT_Checklist_PDF_Fillable_Form.pdf
8. Three questions on the CASP checklist for critically appraising qualitative studies:

Are the results of the study valid?
What are the results?
Will the results help locally?

EXERCISE 4: CONDUCTING CRITICAL APPRAISALS TO BUILD AN EVIDENCE-BASED PRACTICE

Notes for Critical Appraisal of Steffen et al. (2021) Study

1. Writing quality: Overall, the Steffen et al. (2021) research report was well organized, detailed, and clearly written.
2. Title: Interesting and identified the intervention of the RCT and population.
3. Abstract: Clear, concise coverage of the study design, participants, intervention, outcomes, key results, and conclusions.
4. Problem: Serious worldwide health problem of managing people with type 2 diabetes mellitus (T2DM) and associated arterial hypertension (AH). People affected have high morbidity and mortality. The care of people with chronic conditions is "generally inefficient, unsystematic, prescriptive, rushed, and with lack of dignity for the patients" (problem statement; Steffen et al., 2021, p. e204).
5. Purpose: Concisely stated, addressed the problem statement, and directed the study methodology.
6. Review of literature: Adequate coverage of the empirical literature for the motivational interviewing (MI) intervention. No coverage of the outcomes measures, hemoglobin (HbA1c) and blood pressure BP). Theoretical literature was not noted.
7. Framework: Chronic Care Model was mentioned as the basis for the risk strata used to identify the study population but was not identified as the study framework. Thus, the study lacked an identified framework, which limits the link of the framework to the operational definitions of the variables and the link of study findings to the nursing body of knowledge.
8. Objects, questions, or hypotheses: None were stated for this study. Hypotheses were needed to test the propositions from the framework, direct the study methodology, and organized the research results.
9. Variables: MI intervention, HbA1c, and BP lacked conceptual definitions but had clear, relevant operational definitions.

10. Research design: The design was clearly identified (parallel-group RCT), which is considered one of the strongest quantitative designs. Participants were randomized into the intervention and usual care groups. Blinding was implemented related to measurement of the outcome variables and data analysis. The methodology followed the international standard for conducting RCT (CONSORT, 2010). The CONSORT flow diagram was included in the study report.
11. Sample: A power analysis was conducted to determine sample size but the ideal sample size (248) was not research due to lack of resources. A total of 174 participants completed the study. The smaller sample size reduced the power of the study and probably resulted in a Type II error, because the HbA1c results were not significantly different between the intervention and usual care groups.
12. Protection of human subjects: The study was managed ethically with the approval an institutional review board and each participant signing a consent form.
13. The setting was identified and appropriate for the purpose study.
14. MI Intervention was adequately described and the training of the nurses for implementing intervention was detailed. The researchers noted the limitation of the lack of feedback on MI to the nurses during the study, which resulted in a lack of information about intervention fidelity.
15. Measurement: The researchers included limited information about the precision and accuracy of the HbA1c and BP measurements. Limited reliability and validity were provided for the Beck Depression Inventory used to measure depression and the Martín-Bayarre-Grade Questionnaire to measure adherence. Depression and adherence were considered confounding variables with their effects removed statistically.
16. Data collection: The implementation of the MI and the collection of data for HbA1c, BP, depression, and adherence were described.
17. Data analysis: The statistical analyses conducted were clearly identified and appropriate to address the aim of this study. The results were presented concisely in tables and clearly discussed in the study narrative. The results would have been more organized,

clear, and concise if the researchers had developed hypotheses and used these to guide the presentation of the Results section and the discussion of findings.

18. Interpretation of findings: The MI group had significantly lower BPs than the usual care group but no significant difference for HbA1c values. However, the MI group participants showed a 0.4% reduction in HbA1c values ($p < 0.01$). The study findings were described and linked to the findings of previous studies.

19. Limitations: The researchers identified the limitations and the impact they had on the study findings.

20. Conclusions: A separate section addressed conclusions that were appropriate based on the study findings.

21. Nursing implications: MI intervention had potential for use in clinical practice but addition research is recommended first.

22. Further research: Additional quantitative studies were recommended to determine the effectiveness of MI intervention in practice. These studies need a larger, more representative sample; clearly defined HbA1c levels for study participants, and documented intervention fidelity for the MI intervention. Qualitative studies are recommended to determine how nurses providing the intervention and the people receiving it feel about it.

Critical Appraisal Summary for the Steffen et al. (2021) Study

Steffen and colleagues (2021) conducted a quality randomized controlled trial (RCT) according to the international CONSORT (2010)* guidelines. This research report has a focused, interesting title that should catch the attention of many nurses managing patients with type 2 diabetes mellites (T2DM) and associated arterial hypertension (AH). The study abstract includes concise, relevant information about the study design, participants, intervention, outcomes, results, and conclusions. The study problem is also a strength because it addresses a serious worldwide healthcare concern of managing care for individuals with T2DM and AH. These chronic conditions affect millions of people in numerous counties resulting in morbidity, mortality, and excessive costs (American Diabetes Association, 2020; WHO, World Health Statistics, 2018)*. The concisely stated purpose or aim addresses the problem statement and directs the remaining steps of the study.

The review of literature provides adequate coverage of the empirical literature but minimal coverage of theoretical sources. The literature is current with eight of the 44 sources (18.2%) published during the last 5 years and 19 (43.2%) published in the last 10 years. Thus, over 61% of the sources were published in the last 10 years (Grove & Gray, 2023). One of the major weaknesses of the Steffen et al. (2021) study is the lack of theoretical literature and an identified framework to guide the study. The dependent or outcome variables, hemoglobin A1c (HbA1c) and blood pressure (BP) were clearly identified and operationally defined. Motivational interviewing (MI) intervention was also operationally defined but no conceptual definitions were identified for the major study variables. Depression and adherence were clearly identified as confounding variables that were managed statistically during data analysis. This experimental study would have been greatly strengthened by identifying hypotheses based on the relationships in an expressed framework (Grove & Gray, 2023).

The design was one of the strongest aspects of the Steffen et al. (2021) study, which was clearly identified as a parallel-group RCT, one of the strongest experimental designs. The study was ethical with the approval an institutional review board and the participants signing a consent form. Participants were randomized into the intervention and usual care groups. Blinding was implemented with the measurement of the outcome variables and data analysis. The researchers provided a flow diagram (Figure 1) to document the sampling process in their study and identified the attrition as 7 (6.9%) for the intervention group and 8 (9.1%) for the usual care groups. Thus, the attrition was limited and relatively equal for both groups. A power analysis was conducted to determine sample size but the ideal sample size (248) was not achieved due to a lack of resources with only 174 participants completing the study. MI intervention was adequately described as was the training of the nurses implementing the intervention. Steffen et al. (2021) identified relevant limitations that focused on the inadequate sample size and the potential lack of intervention fidelity. The study lacked details about the precision and accuracy of the measures for the HbA1c and BP outcome variables. The scales used to measure depression and adherence did not include adequate reliability and validity information (Grove & Gray, 2023).

---

* Citations from the references of Steffen et al. (2021, pp. e211-e212)

Steffen et al. (2021) provided a detailed discussion of the data collection process. The implementation of the MI intervention and the collection of data for HbA1c, BP, depression, and adherence were clearly presented. The statistical analyses conducted were clearly identified and relevant for the study purpose and the level of measurement of the study variables. The results were concisely presented in tables and clearly discussed in the study narrative.

The Discussion section included an appropriate interpretation of the study findings and a link of those findings with previous study findings. The MI intervention significantly improved the BPs of the intervention group as compared to the usually care group but not the HbA1c. Steffen et al. (2021) reported that the MI had potential for improving the care of individuals with chronic conditions but additional research is needed. They recommend additional quantitative studies with larger more representative samples, participants with abnormal HbA1c, and designated intervention fidelity. Qualitative studies were recommended to determine how nurses providing the intervention and the people receiving it feel about it. In summary, Steffen et al. (2021) conducted a quality study that provided important knowledge for nursing and direction for further research.

Notes for Critical Appraisal of the Colwill et al. (2021) Study

1. Writing quality: Colwill et al. (2021) wrote a clear report, organized into relevant sections. Most of the article was describing the results of the analysis, with numerous quotes from participants. Appropriate for qualitative studies.
2. Title: The researchers included the qualitative method and the sample, but did not indicate the study was about the hospitalizations of persons who inject drugs (PWID).
3. Abstract: *Applied Nursing Research* does not include abstracts for their articles.
4. Research problem: Colwill et al. (2021) noted that hospitalizations of PWID with endocarditis who need surgical intervention had doubled, but did not provide statistics of what the size of the population is. They introduced the ethical dilemma of healthcare providers and the negative perceptions of the public and healthcare providers toward PWID. The problem statement was, "Researchers have not exclusively explored the hospitalized patient perspective in this unique population of PWID with endocarditis as they await a treatment decision" (Colwill et al. 2021, Introduction).

5. Purpose: Develop a model to describe the hospital experiences of PWID with endocarditis. The purpose was congruent with the research problem and guided the study.
6. Literature review: The literature review was primarily reported in the Introduction section. It was concise and focused on the clinical problem and the research problem. Citations were also included in the Discussion to compare the findings with previous research findings.
7. Study framework or philosophical orientation: No framework was identified as is appropriate for a grounded theory study. The researchers alluded to the philosophical orientation, symbolic interaction theory, when they refer to the symbolic meaning of the experiences for PWID.
8. Research objectives (aims) or questions: The research question was clearly stated as "How do PWID hospitalized with endocarditis interpret their lives as they move in and out of the hospital and society?" (Colwill et al., 2021, Methods).
9. Sampling: Although not identified as being the inclusion criteria, participants were PWID with endocarditis in the specific hospital where the study was conducted. The only exclusion criterion was the inability to be interviewed in English. Because the participants were hospitalized for surgical intervention, an exclusion criterion of persons whose physical condition was unstable would have been appropriate. Theoretical purposive sampling was identified, but additional information was not provided about recruiting participants who might provide different perspectives, which is common with theoretical sampling. Potential participants were identified by the primary investigators (JC, MS) from the list of surgical patients with endocarditis.
10. Ethical considerations: The study was approved by hospital's IRB and written consent was obtained from study participants. The authors used pseudonyms to protect confidentiality, but sample characteristics were provided for each participant. The unique combination of characteristics could make the individuals identifiable by nurses who were involved in their care.
11. Data collection: The 11 individual interviews were 7 to 31 minutes in length. Theoretical saturation was reached after the 8th participant. The researchers conducted 3 more

interviews to confirm the core concept. The digitally-recorded interviews were transcribed verbatim by a member of the research team. The lengths of the interviews were shorter than expected but the topic was focused and the participants were persons who were hospitalized with serious illness.

12. Data analysis: The researchers followed the grounded theory methods developed by Straus and Corbin (1998). Data was analyzed concurrently with the interviews. The researchers reported using open, axial, and selective coding at different stages of the analysis. These are types of coding that are consistent with grounded theory. They also clearly described how they resolved differences among team members. The model underwent 20 iterations before it was finalized.

13. Results: Model (Fig.1) developed for the cyclic experiences of hospitalized PWID with endocarditis. The interrelated cycles of The Person and The Healthcare System were displayed inside a circle labeled Society. Each theme had emerged from sub-themes that were supported by multiple quotes of the participants.

Theme	Sub-themes
The person	Want to die, loss of control, withdrawal
The healthcare System	Second chance, desire to live, locus of control
Society	Relationships, trauma and pain, second class citizens, fear, unmet needs

The themes emerged repeatedly in the interviews. The researchers used the recordings and transcripts during the analysis of the data.

14. Interpretation of findings: Endocarditis pushed the PWID into the healthcare system. The themes that had been found in other studies were identified with the appropriate citations (loss of control, locus of control, second class citizen, trauma, unmet needs) as well as the themes that were unique to the study (endocarditis as a catalyst, death, withdrawal, second chance, desire to live, relationships, fear).

15. Limitations: The researchers noted that the study had a small sample size as is typical for qualitative studies and was limited to hospitalized PWID treated in one system in one city. PWID who are not hospitalized may describe their experiences differently. The researchers reiterated that thematic saturation was reached despite small sample size and the methods were rigorous implemented.

16. Conclusions: Greene and Ramos (2021) noted that, as far as they could determine, the model generated during the study was the first person-centered model of PWID with endocarditis being evaluated for surgery. The study provided increased understanding of the thoughts and feelings of PWID who are hospitalized that is the foundation for person-centered care; stigma, both overt and covert, must be identified, addressed, and removed. PWID are vulnerable in multiple ways and need to be treated in comprehensive systems that recognize their personal and social needs.

17. Nursing Implications: More effective interactions and therapeutic communication is possible with increased awareness of the needs of this population. Shows the needed for person-centered care.

18. Future research: Additional studies are needed to develop optional care paths for PWID who have endocarditis. Additional qualitative studies are needed to provide opportunities for stigmatized persons to describe their care needs.

19. Quality of the study: Colwill et al. (2021) identified how their methods supported rigor and produced findings that were confirmable, dependable, credible, and transferable. Confirmability was supported by the constant comparison and team discussions during the analysis. The transcription of the interviews and the review of the results by a drug addiction counselor were identified as methods that supported dependability. The interviewers used a script to ensure the grand tour question was asked consistently in each interview. The interviewers were trained by experienced qualitative researchers and follow-up questions were rehearsed, actions that increase the credibility of the study. The study participants had a wide range of life experiences making the results transferable to other groups of PWID and specifically, those who are hospitalized for surgical evaluation.

Critical Appraisal Summary for the Colwill et al. (2021) Study

Colwill et al. (2021) conducted a grounded theory study with a vulnerable population, using methods developed by recognized experts in qualitative research, Strauss and Corbin (1998).* The title described the qualitative methodology and the population but did not clarify that the participants were hospitalized and being evaluated for surgery. There was no study abstract, which is the practice of the *Applied Nursing Research* journal. The statement of the research problem was clear and the significance of the problem was supported by the growth in the number of hospitalizations for this population in the past 10 years. However, Colwill et al. (2021) did not provide the number of persons living with the diagnosis in the country or the cost of the hospitalization. The stigma of healthcare providers toward PWID and the ethical dilemmas experienced in caring for PWID were mentioned. The results of the study made clear the significance of the problem in terms of suffering and stigmatization of PWID who were hospitalized with endocarditis. The purpose focused on the desired outcome of a model and directed the remaining steps of the study. The research question and the purpose were congruent with each other and were explicitly addressed throughout the study.

The literature review was short, but included two highly relevant studies that were the impetus for the study. Additional sources were cited in the Methods and Discussion sections. Of the 25 references that were cited, 17 (68%) were published in the past 5 years and 6 (24%) were published in the past 6 to 10 years. The remaining two references were the Strauss and Corbin (1998) book on grounded theory and a paper published in 2009 on the ethical decisions of surgeons related to noncompliant patients. The cited studies and other references were relevant and exceptionally current.

The grounded theory method was not linked to a philosophical orientation, but Colwill et al. (2021) referred indirectly to symbolic interaction theory in the discussion when they mentioned the symbolic meaning of the results. Sampling criteria did not mention excluding PWID who were medically unstable. Because all the participants were hospitalized with endocarditis, the length of the interviews was probably appropriate. In addition, the relatively short interviews produced rich data from which 11 sub-themes and 3 interdependent cycles were identified.

The confidentiality of the participants was protected by using pseudonyms. There was a possible threat to confidentiality because the participants were described individually on Table 1. The review by the hospital IRB and the use of written consent forms were actions taken to protect the rights of the participants.

The model produced was complex and included all the sub-themes and endocarditis as the catalyst that moved the Person into the Healthcare System. The title given was "PWID with Endocarditis Cyclical Experiences (PEaCE) model" that described as "a visual representation of the core concept of cyclical life experiences" (Colwill et al., 2021, Summary of the Findings). Some of the sub-themes were supported by the findings of previous studies and others were unique to this study, which expands nursing knowledge related to the care of PWID who have endocarditis. Colwill et al. (2021) identified the limitation of the study being conducted in one location, which raised the question of whether PWID in other parts of the country have similar experiences.

During the data analysis, the researchers enacted several strategies to enhance the rigor of the study, such as conducting the analysis by listening to the recordings and reading the transcripts. Confirmability was supported by the constant comparison and team discussions during the analysis. The transcription of the interviews and the review of the results by a drug addiction counselor were identified as methods that supported dependability. The interviewers used a script to ensure the grand tour question was asked consistently in each interview. The interviewers were trained by experienced qualitative researchers and follow-up questions were rehearsed, actions that increased the credibility of the study. The study participants had a wide range of life experiences making the results transferable to other groups of PWID and specifically, those who are hospitalized for surgical evaluation.

Consistent with the findings, the conclusions were that the study increased nurses' understanding of the thoughts and feelings of PWID with endocarditis hospitalized for surgical evaluation. The potential of being evaluated as not being appropriate for corrective surgery was one indication of the vulnerability of PWID. The researchers identified the need for more effective interactions and therapeutic communication based on an increased awareness of the needs of this population. Person-centered care will only be possible when caregivers are aware of the covert and overt stigma experienced by PWID. Additional quantitative studies are needed to describe and test alternative care paths for PWID who have endocarditis and additional qualitative studies are needed to provide opportunities for stigmatized persons to describe their care needs.

---

* Citations from the references of Colwill et al. (2021, References)

CHAPTER 13—BUILDING AN EVIDENCE-BASED NURSING PRACTICE

EXERCISE 1: TERMS AND DEFINITIONS

Evidence-Based Practice Terms and Research Syntheses
1. f
2. a
3. j
4. b
5. e
6. i
7. h
8. d
9. g
10. k
11. c

Evidence-Based Practice Models
1. b
2. a
3. c
4. b
5. c
6. a

EXERCISE 2: LINKING IDEAS
1. Evidence-based nursing practice promotes desired outcomes for patients, nurses, and healthcare agencies. You might have identified any of the following benefits (or others) for nurses to implement evidence-based practice (EBP).
   a. Improves quality of care delivered by nurses in a variety of healthcare settings.
   b. Improves patient outcomes such as decreased signs and symptoms, improved functional status, improved physical and psychological health, prevention of illnesses, and promotion of health through implementation of healthy lifestyles.
   c. Promotes the delivery of safe care.
   d. Promotes the delivery of cost-effective care.
   e. Decreases need for healthcare services.
   f. Decreases patient recovery time.
   g. Improves the work environment for nurses, increases their productivity, and promotes quality outcomes for patients and nurses.
   h. Accomplishes a Quality and Safety Education for Nurses (QSEN) competency focused on promoting EBP for nursing programs and students.
   i. Increases patient and family satisfaction with care.
   j. Important to meet accreditation requirements.
   k. Important for a healthcare agency to achieve Magnet status.
   l. Increases access to care by providing several types of healthcare agencies and services with a variety of healthcare providers.

2. You might have identified any of the following:
   a. Read research journals in nursing and other healthcare disciplines.
   b. Read clinical journals that have a major focus on publishing research articles.
   c. Use evidence-based websites, such as the Agency for Healthcare Research and Quality (AHRQ) and many others that communicate evidence-based guidelines and reference a variety of research publications. (Table 13.1, Evidence-Based Practice Resources, in Chapter 13 of your textbook, *Understanding Nursing Research*, 8th edition, identifies several resources.)
   d. Attend professional nursing meetings and conferences to obtain information on current studies, research syntheses, and evidence-based guidelines for practice.
   e. Attend nursing research conferences for current study findings and to promote collaboration in research activities.
   f. Participate in collaborative groups of nurses and other healthcare professionals that share research findings in your clinical agencies.
   g. Note study findings reported on television and the Internet and compare the findings to the peer-reviewed report of the study.
   h. Read research findings reported in newspapers and popular journals.
3. You might have identified any of the following challenges to EBP in nursing:
   a. Nursing lacks the research evidence in certain areas for the implementation of EBP.
   b. There is a concern that research evidence generated based on population data might not transfer to the care of individual patients who respond in unique ways.
   c. The best research evidence is currently generated mainly from quantitative and outcomes research methodologies, and more work is needed to synthesize qualitative and mixed methods studies to determine their contributions to EBP.
   d. Some research evidence lacks translation for use in practice.
   e. Healthcare agencies and administrators do not provide the resources to support the implementation of EBP by nurses.
   f. Healthcare agencies and administrators do not provide the resources or support nurses need to participate in research essential to achieve and maintain Magnet status.

4. You might have identified any of the following:
   a. EBP requires the synthesis of research evidence from randomized controlled trials, and these types of studies are limited in nursing.
   b. Researchers have found limited association between nursing interventions/processes and patient outcomes in acute care settings.
   c. There is significant variation in the methods to measure the effect of independent variables (nursing interventions) on patient outcomes.
   d. There is a need for additional studies to determine the effectiveness of nursing interventions.
   e. More replication studies are needed to strengthen the knowledge in significant areas of nursing practice.
   f. There is a need to identify areas where research evidence is needed for practice.
   g. Nurses need to be more active in conducting quality syntheses (systematic reviews, meta-analyses, meta-syntheses, and mixed methods research syntheses) of research evidence in selected areas.

5. You might have identified any two of the following methods for integrating and sustaining a practice change.
   a. Identify and engage key personnel
   b. Hardwire or incorporate the practice change into the healthcare system (revise policies and procedures to be consistent with the needed evidence-based practice change)
   c. Monitor key indicators through quality improvement
   d. Reinfuse or provide education and training as needed to support the practice change

6. Ways research findings might be translated or applied into nursing practice:
   a. Immediate use—using research-based intervention in practice exactly as it was developed.
   b. Reinvention—occurs when the research intervention is modified to meet the needs of a healthcare agency or nurses within the agency.
   c. Cognitive change—occurs when nurses incorporate research findings into their knowledge bases and use this information to defend a point, write/revise agency protocols or policies, or develop a clinical paper for presentation or publication.

7. Formal and informal evaluations of outcomes for the following groups:
   a. patients, families, and communities
   b. nurses and other healthcare professionals
   c. administrators and healthcare agencies

8. feasibility, current practice
9. translation of research evidence into practice, development of evidence-based guidelines, or the use of evidence-based guidelines in practice.
10. Evidence-Based Practice Centers (EPCs)

Understanding Research Syntheses

1.	d	9.	a,b,c,d
2.	a,b,c,d	10.	c
3.	c	11.	d
4.	a	12.	b
5.	a, b	13.	c
6.	c	14.	a,b,c,d
7.	a	15.	a,b
8.	b		

Application of the Phases of Stetler's Model

1.	c	4.	b
2.	d	5.	e
3.	a		

Application of the Iowa Model of Evidence-Based Practice

1.	e	4.	f
2.	c	5.	d
3.	a	6.	b

Agency's Readiness for Evidence-Based Practice

Obtain the answers to these questions by gathering information in the agency where you are doing your clinical hours this semester. Ask your faculty if these questions might be covered in class or through the online discussion board.

1. Review some of the protocols, algorithms, policies, and guidelines in the unit where you are doing clinical and note if these protocols are documented with research sources. If these documents are without references, you cannot assume they are based on current research. Look up any references that are cited on these practice documents to determine their origin. Have there been additional studies done that are relevant?

2. The policies, protocols, algorithms, and guidelines might be based on the knowledge and experience of the nurses developing them and research articles, but not documented with research references or evidence-based websites.

3. Are there nurses in the agency who are responsible for developing and revising policies, protocols, algorithms, and guidelines, and educating nurses to make the necessary changes in practice? Is there a team of nurses working toward meeting accreditation and Magnet status criteria? These individuals are often the change

agents in an agency and promote the use of evidence-based protocols, algorithms, policies, and guidelines in practice.

4. Ask the staff about access to a library or online research publications in their agency. Do they have Internet access or hard copies of journals, and what are the names of the journals? Are these research journals and/or clinical journals with research articles? Do the nurses have access to evidence-based websites on the computers in their agency?

5. Read the mission and goals of the clinical agency. Ask nurses about the goal of EBP in their agency. What steps have been taken to promote EBP?

6. The healthcare agencies that currently have Magnet status can be viewed online at the American Nurses Credentialing Center (ANCC) website at https://www.nursingworld.org/organizational-programs/magnet/find-a-magnet-organization/. Look on this website for the status of the agency. If the agency has Magnet status, how do they document the outcomes of care in their agency to maintain this status? If the agency is seeking Magnet status, where are they in the process of obtaining this designation? Having Magnet status indicates the agency has a commitment to EBP and excellence in nursing care.

7. "The aim [purpose] of this study was to assess a demonstration project intended to pilot and evaluate a structured EBP education with mentoring innovation for nurses in a multi-hospital system" (Friesen et al., 2017, p. 22). You might share this source with nurses in the clinical agencies where you are completing clinical hours.

EXERCISE 3: WEB-BASED INFORMATION AND RESOURCES

1. Quality and Safety Education for Nurses (QSEN) Institute that includes QSEN competencies: Definition and pre-*licensure knowledge, skills, and attitudes (KSAs)*.

2. *QSEN website is:* http://qsen.org/competencies/pre-licensure-ksas/

3. You might identify any three of the following competencies in the EBP Skills area:
Participate effectively in appropriate data collection and other research activities
Adhere to Institutional Review Board (IRB) guidelines
Base individualized care plan on patient values, clinical expertise, and evidence
Read original research and evidence reports related to area of practice
Locate evidence reports related to clinical practice topics and guidelines

Participate in structuring the work environment to facilitate integration of new evidence into standards of practice
Question rationale for routine approaches to care that result in less-than-desired outcomes or adverse events
Consult with clinical experts before deciding to deviate from evidence-based protocols

4. ONS EBP guidelines for managing anorexia in patients with cancer: https://www.ons.org/pep/anorexia

5. Cochrane Library can be accessed at http://www.cochrane.org and then search for research reviews.

6. CNCF Cochran Resources in Nursing website is: http://nursingcare.cochrane.org/resources

7. Yes, this site does include podcasts at https://nursing.cochrane.org/resources/podcasts

8. NRC Patient Education Reference Center website is: https://www.ebscohost.com/nursing/products/patient-education-reference-center

9. U.S. Preventive Services Task Force Recommendations: Information for Health Professionals' website is: https://www.uspreventiveservicestaskforce.org/uspstf/recommendation-topics/tools-and-resources-for-better-preventive-care

10. The National Institute for Health and Clinical Excellence (NICE) was organized in the United Kingdom and can be accessed at https://www.evidence.nhs.uk/. This site includes access to many health-related guidelines.

11. You can search the Joanna Briggs Institute at https://joannabriggs.org/.

12. The Joanna Briggs Institute is an international evidence-based organization in Australia that provides access to numerous evidence-based healthcare syntheses, summaries, guidelines, and other EBP resources.

EXERCISE 4: CONDUCTING CRITICAL APPRAISALS TO BUILD AN EVIDENCE-BASED PRACTICE

1. Problem statement: "Continued efforts must be made to collect and analyze data regarding the effects of the pandemic on the mental health problems of healthcare workers to obtain a full picture of this phenomenon. Therefore, updated evidence that estimates the global mental health situation among healthcare workers during the COVID-19 pandemic remains necessary" (Saragih et al., 2021, Introduction section).

2. "The authors aimed to provide updated estimates of the prevalence of anxiety, depression, distress, and post-traumatic stress

disorder among healthcare workers during the COVID-19 pandemic" (Saragih et al., 2021, Introduction section). This aim was clearly and concisely presented, addressed the problem statement, and directed the methodology of the research synthesis.

3. "We conducted this systematic review and meta-analysis by following the PRISMA (Preferred Reporting Items for Systematic Reviews and Meta-analysis) guidelines (Moher et al., 2009). The protocol for this review has been registered in the International Prospective Register of Systematic Reviews (PROSPERO): CRD42020219211" (Saragih et al., 2021, Material and methods section). This is a strength because the PRISMA format is the internationally recommended format for reporting systematic reviews and meta-analyses. Another strength is that the protocol for this review was registered at the appropriate international site (PROSPERO).

4. Yes, the PICOS format was included as indicated by the following quote: "The inclusion criteria were determined according to the PICOS method (Population, Issue of interest, Comparison, Outcome, and Study design) (Liberati et al., 2009). The following eligibility criteria were applied: a) professional workers who served as healthcare workers during the COVID-19 pandemic, including physicians, nurses, midwives, paramedics, and other related professional medical workers; b) cohort studies, case–control studies, or cross-sectional studies; and c) published in the English language" (Saragih et al., 2021, Eligibility criteria section). The eligibility criteria for this research synthesis were clearly designated using the PICOS format. The PICOS elements were clearly presented and relevant to the research synthesis conducted.

5. Yes, a rigorous literature search was conducted as indicated by the following quote: "To locate all relevant studies, specific keywords and Medical Subject Heading (MeSH) terms were used to search the following databases: PubMed, Academic Search Complete, Cumulative Index to Nursing and Allied Health Literature (CINAHL), Web of Science, MEDLINE Complete, and socINDEX databases. The literature search was performed from December 1, 2019, to November 2, 2020, with the assistance of a health science librarian.... The search strategy was described in detail in Supplementary Document 1" (Saragih et al., 2021, Search strategy section). Many databases were searched using specific, relevant key words

with the assistance of a librarian. The timeframe for the search was identified and appropriate for the topic of this research synthesis. The authors documented their search strategy for readers to review online.

6. Research reports identified, screened, and included in the research synthesis. The answers to the following questions are presented in Fig. 1 and in the Search results section of the article.
   a. "The search yielded a total of 1046 studies" (Saragih et al., 2021, Search results section).
   b. A total of 526 reports were removed because they were duplicates. This indicates that researchers are publishing duplicates of their work in separate places. Often the original publications are not cited in later publications and are too similar to or the same as the original publication. Duplicate publications are an example of research misconduct (see Chapter 4 in Grove & Gray, 2023).
   c. A total of 38 articles underwent full-text review.
   d. The systematic review included 38 studies. The selection process for these 38 studies is detailed in a PRISMA Flow Diagram (Fig. 1) and in the article's narrative in the Search results section.

7. A meta-analysis was conducted for each of the mental health problems to determine the prevalence of anxiety, depression, distress, and post-traumatic stress disorder in healthcare workers globally during the COVID-19 pandemic. The meta-analysis results are presented in Fig. 2, Fig. 3, Fig. 4, and Fig. 5.

8. A 49% prevalence of post-traumatic stress disorder was found in the healthcare workers. This was the most common mental health problem identified.

9. Assessment of the studies' quality included: "The 8-questions of the Joanna Briggs Institute tool for cross-sectional studies and the 10-questions of the Joanna Briggs Institute tool for case–control studies were used to appraise the study's quality for 38 included studies. Three studies scored 8 out of 8 among the 37 studies assessed with the Joanna Briggs Institute tool for cross-sectional studies, 20 studies scored 7 out of 8, 13 studies scored 6 out of 8, and four studies scored 5 out of 8. ... All of the scores for the assessed studies indicate a low risk of bias" (Saragih et al., 2021, Quality assessment section). A structured assessment of the studies' quality was conducted and clearly presented in tables. A summary of the characteristics of the 38 studies was detailed in Table 1.

10. Conclusions: "In summary, we aimed to study the prevalence of mental health problems among healthcare workers during the COVID-19 pandemic. We showed that the most prevalent mental health disorder experienced by healthcare workers was post-traumatic stress disorder, followed by anxiety, depression, and distress" (Saragih et al., 2021, Conclusion section).

11. "Future studies remain necessary to assess the factors associated with the development of mental health problem among healthcare workers during COVID-19. The global COVID-19 pandemic has placed the physical health of healthcare workers at the highest risk of being infected by the virus. The global population has responsibility for healing their healers, establishing a resilient work-force environment, and respecting their totality. Strong recommendations are aimed at governments, policy-makers, and relevant stakeholders to pay close attention to and address the mental health burdens of health care workers. Specific interventional research is urgently necessary to mitigate the mental health impacts on healthcare workers and to help them cope with their burdens" (Saragih et al., 2021, Conclusion section).

Additional Evidence-Based Practice Projects

1. Use the content in Chapter 13 of your textbook, *Understanding Nursing Research*, 8th edition, to implement an EBP project guided by Stetler's Model (textbook Figure 13.2) or the Iowa Evidence-Based Model (textbook Figure 13.3).
2. Use the Grove Model in textbook Fig. 13.4 to direct the implementation of the evidence-based guidelines.

CHAPTER 14—INTRODUCTION TO ADDITIONAL RESEARCH METHODOLOGIES IN NURSING: MIXED METHODS AND OUTCOMES RESEARCH

Introduction to Mixed Methods Research

EXERCISE 1: TERMS AND DEFINITIONS FOR MIXED METHODS RESEARCH

1. d
2. a
3. c
4. e
5. b

EXERCISE 2: LINKING IDEAS FOR MIXED METHODS RESEARCH

Key Ideas for Mixed Methods Research

1. The answers could be any of the following:
   a. Mixed methods studies often require a team of researchers with different backgrounds and abilities. Developing a proposal with a team may require more time to come to agreement on a research plan.
   b. For some designs, one phase of the study must be completed and the data analyzed before the second phase is implemented, which requires additional time.
   c. Mixed methods studies often involve more data to be analyzed, requiring more time.
   d. Two types of data must be analyzed and then integrated for an additional level of meaning.
2. quantitative
3. Parallel design
4. Correct answers are any of the following:
   a. The research topic is relevant and significant.
   b. The rationale for using a mixed methods study design was adequate and clear.
   c. The specific mixed methods study design was identified.
   d. The qualitative approach was appropriate for the research question.
   e. The participants recruited for the qualitative phase were recruited appropriately.
   f. The qualitative data were collected and analyzed appropriately.
   g. The researchers described the actions they took to ensure the accuracy of the data transcription and analysis.
   h. The researchers provided participants' quotes to substantiate the themes or main ideas emerging from the analysis.
   i. The strengths and weaknesses of the qualitative phase were identified.
   j. The participants for the quantitative phase were recruited appropriately.
   k. If there was an intervention in the quantitative phase, intervention fidelity was discussed.
   l. The measurement methods were reliable and valid.
   m. Appropriate statistical analyses were used to answer the research questions.
   n. The strengths and weaknesses of the quantitative phase were identified.
   o. If the design is a sequential one, the results of the first phase analysis and its interpretation were used to refine the methods of the second phase.

p. If a concurrent design was used, the results of the two phases were integrated and interpreted to produce the findings.

q. The contributions to knowledge that were made by conducting a mixed methods study were identified.

r. The strengths and weaknesses of the study were identified.

5. Compare what you drew to Fig. 14.3 (Grove & Gray, 2023). The qualitative phase should be shown first followed by data analysis and interpretation prior to the quantitative phase of the study.

6. The quantitative phase would have been shown first followed by data analysis and interpretation prior to the qualitative phase of the study.

Mixed Methods Research Methodologies

1. b. (quantitative followed by qualitative)
2. b. (quantitative followed by qualitative)
3. a. (quantitative and qualitative at the same time)
4. c. (qualitative followed by quantitative)
5. a. (quantitative and qualitative at the same time)

EXERCISE 3: WEB-BASED INFORMATION AND RESOURCES FOR MIXED METHODS RESEARCH

1. https://obssr.od.nih.gov/research-resources/mixed-methods-research
2. Creswell, Klassen, Clark, and Smith
3. https://www.scribbr.com/methodology/mixed-methods-research/
4. Scribbr
5. https://publichealth.jhu.edu/academics/academic-programs/training-grants/mixed-methods-research-training-program-for-the-health-sciences

EXERCISE 4: CONDUCTING CRITICAL APPRAISALS TO BUILD AN EVIDENCE-BASED PRACTICE

Mixed Methods Research

1. The relevance and significance of the topic was clearly described in the first paragraph and supported by citing several studies about the importance of the patient-provider trust. Patient-provider trust is related to an effective provider-patient relationship, better health behaviors, utilization of services, more engaged patients, patients' likelihood of following provider recommendations, and better control of chronic conditions. Patient-provider trust is also related to adhering to appointments and seeking care when needed.

2. Greene and Ramos (2021) identified different ways that trust between patients and providers had been measured, but noted that trust had been conceptualized in different ways. They inferred the differences in conceptual definitions was the motivation for using qualitative and quantitative methods to study the research topic. The researchers did not clearly state their rationale.

3. Exploratory sequential mixed methods design

4. The researchers used the findings of the qualitative data collection and analysis to select items to be analyzed from the Health Reform Monitoring Survey (HRMS).

5. Yes, but the researchers did not call them contributions to knowledge. You may have identified any of the following as contributions. The first was their primary finding: "These three dimensions of trust [communication, caring, competence], which were identified through qualitative interviews, were found to be highly correlated with trust in a recent national survey, and were consistently related to trust regardless of participants' race/ethnicity or income" (Greene & Ramos, 2021, p. 1226). Another contribution was that the study's participants described trust differently than how most instruments measured the concept. The researchers found only one instrument that measured all three of the dimensions of trust identified in the qualitative phase, and that instrument was long and measured unrelated concepts. The findings provide a framework for future studies.

6. One of the weaknesses was that the participants in the qualitative component were disproportionately vulnerable. The researchers explained why they did this and that the quantitative results indicated no differences based on race/ethnicity nor income. Minimal detail was provided about the HRMS national survey and the quality of the data collected. In addition, the design of the quantitative part of this mixed methods study lacked detail. Another limitation was that the researchers could not test every aspect of their qualitative findings. Another limitation was that they measured interpersonal trust between patient and providers, not other aspects of trust that may be important such as trust in health care in general. One strength was that the findings indicate ways that providers could encourage their patients to trust them. The study used a relatively large sample for the qualitative component and quantitative data from a national study sample.

7. Greene and Ramos (2021) conducted an exploratory sequential mixed methods study of the trust between patients and providers. The topic was significant because trust had been shown in previous studies to be linked to patient engagement and health outcomes. The researchers could have been clearer on the rationale for using a mixed methods design. The participants in both components of the study had participated in the national survey of the HRMS and indicated they had a usual healthcare provider. Participants in the qualitative component also indicated they were willing to be contacted for a telephone interview. The participants in the quantitative component were those who had complete data on the identified variables. The length of the telephone interviews was shorter than most interviews, but produced rich data. The data analysis and interpretation revealed findings that added to what is known about trust. In addition, a framework was developed that can be used in future studies. Study limitations included being unable to test all aspects of the qualitative findings and focusing only on trust between patient and provider. These limitations are due to using an existing dataset, which can also be viewed as a strength because of the large sample size. Greene and Ramos (2021) conducted a rigorous mixed methods study that can serve as a starting point for future studies.

Introduction to Outcomes Research

EXERCISE 1: TERMS AND DEFINITIONS FOR OUTCOMES RESEARCH

1.	f	7.	e
2.	h	8.	l
3.	g	9.	k
4.	a	10.	c
5.	d	11.	j
6.	i	12.	b

EXERCISE 2: LINKING IDEAS FOR OUTCOMES RESEARCH

Key Ideas for Outcomes Research

1. Avedis Donabedian
2. Aspects of person or patient health:
   a. Physical–psychological function
   b. Psychological function
   c. Social function

3. Your examples may be any of the answers listed for each foci or others you might identify.
   a. Structure: Nursing units, hospitals, clinics, or home health agencies; types of providers such as physicians and nurse practitioners; patient characteristics
   b. Process: Focused on the care that is provided or practice patterns of interventions in managing patients. How the care is provided or practice style and standards of care delivered (clinical guidelines, critical paths, or care maps)
   c. Outcomes: Morbidity and mortality rates, length of stay in healthcare agencies, complications from procedures, side effects of medications, medication errors, fall rates, infection rates, and costs; patient signs and symptoms, functional status, psychological health, and patient satisfaction
4. assessment, nursing diagnosis, nurse-initiated interventions, and follow-up care
5. communication, case management, coordination of care, continuity/monitoring, and reporting
6. process of care
7. Standards of care
   a. Clinical guidelines
   b. Critical paths
   c. Care maps
8. heterogeneous
9. You might have listed any of the following questions:
   a. What are the end results of patients' care (all care provided by all care providers)?
   b. What effects does nursing care (all care by all nurses) have on the end results of patients care?
   c. Are there some nursing acts that have no effect at all on outcomes or that cause harm?
   d. Can we measure and thus identify the end results of nursing care?
   e. How do we distinguish care provided by nurses from care provided by other professionals in examining patient outcomes?
   f. When do we measure the effects of care (end results) (e.g., change in symptoms, functioning, or quality of life): immediately after the care, when the patient is discharged, or much later?
10. Types of databases
    a. Administrative
    b. Clinical

11. Nursing Outcomes Classification (NOC)
12. change; improvement
13. Major questions to critically appraise outcome studies
    a. What are the results?
    b. Are the results valid?
    c. How can I apply the results to patient care?

Outcomes Research Methodologies

1. d
2. c
3. e
4. b
5. a

EXERCISE 3: WEB-BASED INFORMATION AND RESOURCES FOR OUTCOMES RESEARCH

1. Agency for Healthcare Research and Quality AHRQ website: http://www.ahrq.gov/research/index.html
2. Patient-Centered Outcomes Research Institute (PICORI)
3. PICORI website: https://www.pcori.org/
4. Vision & Mission of PICORI website: https://www.pcori.org/about-us/our-vision-mission
5. Vision: Patients and the public have information they can use to make decisions that reflect their desired health outcomes. Mission: PCORI helps people make informed healthcare decisions, and improves healthcare delivery and outcomes, by producing and promoting high-integrity, evidence-based information that comes from research guided by patients, caregivers, and the broader healthcare community.
6. National Quality Forum (NQF) Website: https://www.qualityforum.org/home.aspx
7. National Database of Nursing Quality Indicator website: http://www.nursingquality.org/
8. American Nurses Association (ANA)
9. Your answer will depend on which website you selected. YouTube videos start with https://www.youtube.com/watch. Compare your answers with those of your peers to identify helpful videos. Examples of URLs on nurse sensitive outcomes or indicators include: https://www.youtube.com/watch?v=91eM3yElZu4 and https://www.youtube.com/watch?v=Ot_-5vZV6lI
10. Website Nursing Outcomes Classification (NOC): http://www.nursing.uiowa.edu/cncce/nursing-outcomes-classification-overview

EXERCISE 4: CONDUCTING CRITICAL APPRAISALS TO BUILD AN EVIDENCE-BASED PRACTICE

Outcomes Research

The critical appraisal is of the Jeong et al. (2020) study.

1. Jeong et al. (2020, p. 741) reported the following problem and purpose for their study: "Racial disparities in quality of life and health outcomes among nursing home residents have been well documented, particularly in the United States. However, no studies, to our knowledge, have assessed the association between immigrant status and health outcomes of nursing home residents. In this study, we aimed to (1) describe the characteristics of immigrants entering nursing homes, and (2) compare hospitalization and mortality rates of immigrants and long-term residents in their first year of living in a nursing home."
2. A population-based retrospective cohort study was conducted. The population was nursing home residents and the data were obtained from health administrative databases.
3. Yes, the outcomes research methods implemented in the study were clearly identified in the title of the article and in the Methods section. The Methods section addressed the study problem and purpose.
4. The outcome variables examined in the study included: hospitalizations, emergency department visits, mortality, intensive care visits, and location of death. The researchers examined the rates of all outcomes within the first year of each resident's nursing home admission.
5. Location of death was operationally defined as acute care (including hospitals and emergency departments), nursing home, or other.
6. Yes, a secondary data analysis was conducted with health administrative databases.
7. The outcomes data "were obtained from the Discharge Abstract Database (DAD), National Ambulatory Care Reporting System (NACRS), and RPDB [Registered Persons Database] databases, respectively" (Jeong et al., 2020, p. 741).
8. The sample included 57,115 residents newly admitted to one of 648 Ontario, Canada nursing homes after 1985. There were 2536 (4.4%) immigrants and 54,579 (95.6%) long term Canadian residents. The demographic

and clinical characteristics of the participants were detailed in Tables 1 and 2 of the study to provide a picture of the sample. This study had an extremely large heterogeneous sample, which is a strength in outcomes studies (Grove & Gray, 2023). The sample was appropriate to address the study purpose. Jeong et al. (2020, p. 745) reported: "A major strength of this study was the large, population-based cohort and use of healthcare and administrative data sets linked at the individual level. The linkage allowed us to adjust for many confounding variables such as living arrangements prior to nursing home entry, socioeconomic status reflected through neighborhood income quintiles, and other baseline characteristics."

9. The setting for the Jeong et al. (2020) study was nursing homes in Ontario. Participants from an extensive number of nursing homes (648) were included in the data analysis, which ensured the representativeness of the settings and participants for this Canadian province.

10. Conclusions: "We have demonstrated lower 1-year mortality among immigrants in nursing homes, showing the healthy immigrant effect potentially applies even to the frailest population who requires nursing home care. Immigrants are less likely to enter nursing homes, alluding to differences in preferences and needs. Despite the healthy immigrant effect, immigrants have higher rates of hospitalization in the first year of living in a nursing home. Inability to speak English was associated with increased risk of hospitalization" (Jeong et al., 2020, p. 745).

11. Jeong et al., 2020, p. 745) reported: "the need for strategies to overcome communication barriers. To reduce disparities in access and outcomes, there is a need to support cultural and linguistic diversity in long-term care settings." These implications are appropriate based on the study findings and limitations. They also recommended "future research in this topic would provide greater insight into the impact of culture and language in the health of nursing home residents" (Jeong et al., 2020, p. 745).

12. Critical appraisal: The research problem was significant and addressed by the research purpose. The study purpose was clearly stated, relevant, and directed the methods of this outcomes study. The sample and setting were extremely strong in this study and provided a large heterogenous sample of participants, who were representative of Ontario nursing homes. The study design, population-based retrospective cohort, was clearly identified and appropriate for this study. The data analyses addressed the study purpose and the results were clearly presented in the study narrative and tables. The study limitations were identified, such as the lack of data available on culture factors and relevant confounding variables. The study conclusions were consistent with the study results and findings and addressed the study purpose. The study would have been strengthened by including a framework, such as the Donabedian Model for quality of care that is often used to organize findings obtained from outcome studies.

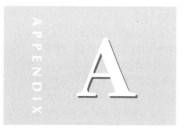

Quantitative Study

American Journal of
Preventive Medicine
RESEARCH ARTICLE

Motivational Interviewing in the Management of Type 2 Diabetes Mellitus and Arterial Hypertension in Primary Health Care: An RCT

Pâmela L.S. Steffen, MSc,[1] Claunara S. Mendonça, PhD,[1] Elisabeth Meyer, PhD,[2]
Daniel D. Faustino-Silva, PhD[1]

Introduction: Motivational interviewing is an effective style of collaborative communication for the promotion of lifestyle changes in the management of Type 2 diabetes and arterial hypertension. This study evaluates the effectiveness of motivational interviewing in the management of these conditions in primary health care.

Study Design: This study is a double-blind parallel-group RCT performed between June 2018 and July 2019.

Setting/participants: The RCT was conducted in Porto Alegre, Rio Grande do Sul, Brazil, and included individuals with Type 2 diabetes and arterial hypertension.

Intervention: The participants were randomized to the test/motivational interviewing and usual care groups. The test/motivational interviewing group received the nursing consultation intervention on the basis of motivational interviewing conducted by professionals with 20 hours of training, and the usual-care group received conventional nursing consultation.

Main outcome measures: The main outcome measure was the mean difference in HbA1c. The secondary outcome measures were the mean differences in blood pressure and adherence levels.

Results: After a mean follow-up of 6 months, 174 participants completed the study (usual-care group=80; test/motivational interviewing group=94). There were statistically significant differences between the groups, with improvement in the test/motivational interviewing group for systolic blood pressure ($p<0.01$), diastolic blood pressure ($p<0.01$), and total adherence score as measured by the Martín−Bayarre−Grade questionnaire ($p=0.01$) and its operational dimensions of treatment adherence and personal involvement ($p=0.03$, $p=0.03$). The test/motivational interviewing group showed significantly reduced HbA1c levels (0.4%) at the end of the study ($p<0.01$).

Conclusions: In the context of primary health care, the nursing consultation based on motivational interviewing was shown to be a more effective care strategy than usual care for improving blood pressure levels and adherence levels in individuals with Type 2 diabetes and arterial hypertension. Moreover, motivational interviewing was demonstrated to be useful in reducing HbA1c levels in diabetes management.

Trial registration: This study is registered at www.clinicaltrials.gov NCT03729323.
Am J Prev Med 2021;60(5):e203−e212. © 2021 American Journal of Preventive Medicine. Published by Elsevier Inc. All rights reserved.

From the [1]Graduate Program in Assessment and Production of Technologies for the SUS (PPGATSUS), Grupo Hospitalar Conceição (GHC), Porto Alegre, Brazil; and [2]Graduate Program in Health Sciences, Instituto de Cardiologia (IC/FUC), Porto Alegre, Brazil

Address correspondence to: Daniel D. Faustino-Silva, PhD, Gerência de Ensino e Pesquisa, Centro Administrativo, Hospital Nossa Senhora da Conceição, 1° andar. Av. Francisco Trein, 596, CEP, Porto Alegre 91350-200, Brazil. E-mail: ddemetrio@gmail.com.

0749-3797/$36.00
https://doi.org/10.1016/j.amepre.2020.12.015

e204   *Steffen et al / Am J Prev Med 2021;60(5):e203—e212*

INTRODUCTION

Type 2 diabetes mellitus (T2DM) is a serious public health problem worldwide. When associated with a diagnosis of arterial hypertension (AH), T2DM has even higher morbidity and mortality, requiring increased efforts in its management. One of the main challenges in preventing, treating, and controlling T2DM and AH is strategizing with the person at the center of care, engaging patients and supporting patients' shared decision making—interventions in which primary care nurses play an important role.[1-8] In particular, the difficulties faced by individuals in adapting their habits to a healthy lifestyle and reconciling their daily activities with the medical treatment and different care technologies has been a gap that requires effective intervention from professionals.

Motivational interviewing (MI) is a collaborative style of communication. Clinical evidence has shown that MI strengthens the person's motivation and commitment to change behaviors in the interest of their health, on the basis of respect for their autonomy. The guiding principles of MI are based on resisting the righting reflex, understanding and exploring the patient's motivations, listening with empathy, and empowering the patient, thus stimulating hope and optimism.[9] In primary care environments, MI is an inexpensive and high-potential impact strategy that can be learned by different categories of health professionals and applied regardless of age, sex, or severity of the patient's health problem.[9-12]

However, despite the promising panorama reflected by the growing number of international studies, research into and dissemination of MI in professional training and practice for the management of T2DM and AH in routine primary health care is still in its early stages.[13,14] The prevailing reality is still that of epidemiologically alarming numbers of chronic conditions with standards of care that are generally inefficient, unsystematic, prescriptive, rushed, and with lack of dignity for the patient.[1,5,6,15,16] The aim of this study is to evaluate the effectiveness of MI in individual nursing consultations for the management of T2DM with AH in the context of primary health care.

METHODS

This was a parallel-group RCT conducted in 3 health units in the *Zona Norte* (North Zone) of Porto Alegre, Rio Grande do Sul, Brazil, between June 2018 and July 2019. The methods followed the recommendations of the CONSORT 2010 information list, and the project was previously registered at clinicaltrials.gov under NCT03729323. Study participants, the person responsible for randomization and allocation, the people responsible for measurement of outcome variables, and those responsible for data analysis were blinded. It was impossible to blind interventionists because of the requirement for training and the procedures necessary to conduct the study.

Study Population

Study participants were individuals with T2DM and an associated diagnosis of AH, were registered in the health units established as the research settings, and were with Risk Strata 3 and 4. Risk strata were based on the stratification model used at those services, which considers the severity of the chronic condition and the patient's self-management capabilities, on the basis of the Chronic Care Model.[17] Risk Stratum 3 is an intermediate stratum in which the disease represents moderate or high cardiovascular risk level according to the Framingham Risk Score, but cardiovascular disease has not been established. Risk Stratum 4 covers the population with a chronic condition of high cardiovascular risk, with or without established complications but with severe difficulties in self-management.

The health units were selected on the basis of the similarity of epidemiologic profile and health indicators in T2DM and AH, being the 3 largest in the *Serviço de Saúde Comunitária do Grupo Hospitalar Conceição* (SSC/GHC) (Community Health Service of the Conceição Hospital Group). The inclusion criteria were being aged ≥18 years, having a medical diagnosis of T2DM associated with AH, and being registered in the programmatic actions of the study units in Risk Strata 3 and 4. The exclusion criteria were refusal to sign the informed consent form, patient not found after 3 attempts to contact by phone or in person at home, and illiteracy or a medical diagnosis of mental and behavioral disorders with impaired mental faculties.[18]

Because of the absence of a pilot study, a study with a similar research protocol was used to anticipate the expected effect size. On the basis of that study, investigators added 10% for possible losses and refusals, and the sample size was estimated at 248 patients by Winpepi, version 11.61. The authors considered a power of 80%, a significance level of 5%, and an SD of 2% for a mean difference of 0.75% in HbA1c.[19]

Measures

Simple individual randomization was performed electronically by the SSC/GHC Monitoring and Evaluation center by a professional who was not part of the study team. The professional randomized and allocated all possible eligible patients into 2 groups—test/MI group and usual-care group—before the research team initiated recruitment. Participants allocated in each group were recruited in ascending order, and if they met the inclusion and acceptance criteria, they were electronically scheduled for the corresponding intervention. Blinded allocation was guaranteed by the protection of randomized lists in an electronic file and respective electronic scheduling system with access restricted to those responsible for recruiting the participants in each research setting. Recruiters were trained community health agents who used a single, standardized invitation model that followed the process of scheduling appointments, without any differentiation between the groups. On acceptance to participate, individuals received at home a brown envelope with the informed consent form and instructions for the start of interventions from the community health agent. At the end of the study, the electronic lists were verified for the

Steffen et al / Am J Prev Med 2021;60(5):e203—e212 e205

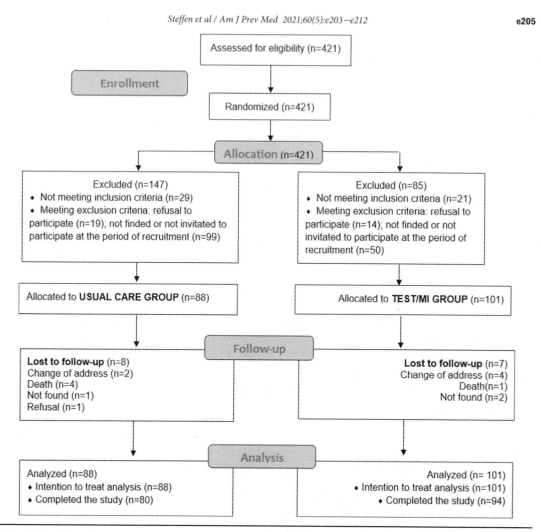

Figure 1. Study flow chart.
MI, motivational interviewing.

purposes of the fidelity test by a professional who was not part of the study team.

Because of the period stipulated for recruitment, some of the eligible patients were not contacted according to their order in the list. Except for patients who were not contacted or who did not meet inclusion criteria/met the exclusion criteria at the time of the recruitment, all patients who consented to participate were analyzed, regardless of whether they received both intervention sessions or had final outcomes collected (Figure 1).

The test/MI group received 2 MI-based nursing consultation sessions lasting 30—50 minutes and conducted monthly by nurses who received 20 hours of training in the use of MI.[10,19] The usual-care group received 2 nursing consultations lasting 30—50 minutes and conducted monthly by professional nurses not trained in the use of MI.[20] The 3 research settings followed the

evidence-based multiprofessional protocol of the SSC/GHC and its regular updates for the organization of the work process and care of people with diabetes and hypertension.

The period between study consultations depended on the patient's health needs and availability. The overall mean time between the first and second nursing consultations was 45 days, with a median of 38 days in the usual-care group and 37 days in the test/MI group. At least 1 telephone call was made to all individuals between the second nursing consultation and the end-of-study call to reinforce what had been agreed on and minimize losses to follow-up.[12]

A total of 8 nurses specializing in public health with ≥5 years of professional experience in primary care were responsible for applying the nursing consultations. Nurses responsible for delivering the nursing consultation to the test/MI group received

May 2021

e206 *Steffen et al / Am J Prev Med 2021;60(5):e203−e212*

intensive training in active learning of basic principles, spirit, and techniques of MI, focusing on the development of empathic communication skills, simple and advanced reflective listening to work on resistance, dealing with ambivalence, exploring discrepancies, and promoting conversation about change.[21] The workshop was conducted by a psychologist member of the study team who has a PhD in psychiatry and extensive experience in conducting MI training workshops for different health segments. The training included didactic presentations and experiential exercises, as recommended by Moyers et al.,[22] with a total work load of 20 hours. Experiential exercises, such as roleplaying, occupied 70% of the total training time, being performed in pairs and, eventually, with a third participant as an observer. The instructor provided feedback on the exercises throughout the training.

Before and after the training, nurses filled out 3 validated questionnaires to assess the importance and confidence in the use of MI and their mastery of the initial basic skills to apply MI in practice: the Importance and Confidence Ruler[21] to use MI; the Conversational Interview Exercise,[21] which identifies the key elements of MI, such as the use of reflections and open-ended questions; and the Helpful Responses Questionnaire,[23] plus MI skills indicators, according to the Motivational Interviewing Skill Code,[24,25] used to assess training effectiveness.

The outcomes were measured at baseline and at 3 months after the second nursing consultation as final outcomes. The measurements were conducted in a blinded form, except for the participant profile questionnaire, which was completed by a nurse during the interventions because it contained important clinical data that required confirmation and updating of these records in the patient's medical records.

The main outcome measure was the mean difference in HbA1c. HbA1c was measured through laboratory tests of blood samples collected in the outpatient department, following the routine practices of these services and without any differentiation between the groups. The secondary outcome measures were the mean differences in blood pressure (BP) measured in the Health Unit by nursing technicians who were not included in the study team; following the routine and technical guidelines inherent to the procedure, without differentiation between the groups[7,26]; and the level of adherence and its dimensions, which was collected using a specific, self-report questionnaire delivered to the participant's home by community health workers. Because of the correlation among adherence, motivation, and depression in chronic diseases, symptoms of depression were measured at baseline as a risk factor for poorer clinical outcomes and therefore were a possible confounder.[7,27]

A semistructured interview for sociodemographic profile and health history instrument was developed by the researchers and contains the variables presented in Table 1.

The Beck Depression Inventory is a self-report and depression screening instrument composed of 21 items, including symptoms and attitudes, in which 20 points is the cut off differentiating a higher level of depressive symptoms.[28,29]

The Martín−Bayarre−Grade Questionnaire is a Cuban questionnaire, but the version used in this study was adapted to the Brazilian context.[30] It is a self-reported questionnaire that determines patients' level of adherence on the basis of the WHO concept of adherence, which includes the adoption of healthy behaviors, personal involvement in the process, and the professional−patient relationship, in addition to taking medication as prescribed.[6,31,32] The questionnaire comprises 12 statements that are answered on a Likert scale with scores of 4−0 points for the responses: *always, almost always, sometimes, almost never,* and *never.*[30] On the basis of the scores given, people are classified as having full adherence, partial adherence, or nonadherence. Moreover, the questionnaire allows for analyzing adherence through its operational dimensions: treatment adherence (i.e., execution and follow-up of prescribed medical indications), personal involvement (i.e., patient search for strategies and efforts necessary to adhere to the prescribed treatment), and patient−therapist relationship (i.e., a collaborative relationship established between the patient and the professional).[30,31]

The study began after submission to and approval by the Research Ethics Committee of the *Grupo Hospitalar Conceição,* under Number 18051 of April 11, 2018. The study complied with Resolution 466/12 of the National Health Council of the Ministry of Health, which deals with research involving human beings, and with the Code of Ethics of Nursing Professionals.[33] After accepting the invitation, all individuals received and signed an informed consent form as a requirement before receiving the interventions.

Statistical Analysis

Researchers used SPSS, version 20.0, for statistical analysis. To assess the normality of continuous variables, the Shapiro−Wilk test was performed. To compare the participants' baseline characteristics, Pearson chi-square test was used and, where necessary, Fisher's exact test and the Student's *t*-test were applied. For the intragroup analysis, the generalized estimating equation model was used, followed by multiple comparisons with Bonferroni correction. For statistical adjustment, because of the significant differences between groups in relation to the baseline variables systolic BP (SBP) and consultation with a nurse in the previous year and because of the influence of the possible confounder of change in pharmacological medical prescription, which could affect the investigated clinical outcomes, ANCOVA was performed for each outcome, considering delta as a dependent variable and the aforementioned variables and baseline values as independent variables. Intention-to-treat analysis was performed, and for dropouts (*n*=15), simple data imputation by last observation carried forward was used. To assess the effect of MI, Cohen's d was applied. The significance level considered for all the analyses was 0.05 (*p*<0.05) with 95% CIs.

RESULTS

Of the 421 eligible randomized and allocated participants, 189 individuals with T2DM and AH were contacted during the recruitment period (June 2018−March 2019), met the inclusion criteria, and agreed to participate. Of these, 174 participants completed the study after a mean time of 6 months between the first consultation and the conclusion of the research protocol with the collection of the final outcomes. Exclusions were based on the inclusion/exclusion criteria. Losses to follow-up were balanced between the groups and were attributed to death, refusal, or delay in collecting the outcomes within the period stipulated for completion of the study and change of address/inability to locate the subject, making

Steffen et al / Am J Prev Med 2021;60(5):e203−e212

Table 1. Comparison of Baseline Sociodemographic and Health History Characteristics of Patients

Variables	Usual care, % (n) (n=88)	Test/MI, % (n) (n=101)	p-value
Sex			0.60[a]
Male	35.2 (31)	41.6 (42)	
Female	64.8 (57)	58.4 (59)	
Age, mean ± SD	66 ± 12	66 ± 8	0.90[b]
Race/ethnicity			0.24[a]
White	83 (73)	78.2 (79)	
Black	14.8 (13)	13.9 (14)	
Mixed	2.3 (2)	7.9 (8)	
Lives alone, yes	20.5 (18)	22.8 (23)	0.53[a]
Education level			0.25[a]
Incomplete primary education	29.5 (26)	21.2 (21)	
Complete primary education	70.5 (62)	78.8 (78)	
Marital status			0.03[a]
Single	17 (15)	9.9 (10)	
Married	50 (44)	54.5 (55)	
Separated/divorced	9.1 (8)	21.8 (22)	
Widow/widower	23.9 (21)	13.9 (14)	
Per capita income[d]			0.27[a]
<1 minimum wage	26.1 (23)	34.7 (34)	
≥1 minimum wage	73.9 (65)	65.3 (64)	
AH diagnosis time, years			0.88[a]
1–5	9.1 (8)	9 (9)	
5–10	21.6 (19)	18 (18)	
>10	69.3 (61)	73 (73)	
T2DM diagnosis time, years			0.17[a]
1–5	26.1 (23)	19.8 (20)	
5–10	27.3 (24)	19.8 (20)	
>10	46.6 (41)	60.4 (61)	
CVD family history, yes	85.9 (73)	90 (90)	0.53[a]
Associated diseases			
CVD	26.1 (23)	27.7 (28)	0.94[a]
Neoplasms	10.2 (9)	10.9 (11)	>0.99[a]
Osteomuscular	8 (7)	24.8 (25)	<0.05[a]
Respiratory tract	9.1 (8)	15.8 (16)	0.24[a]
Diabetic retinopathy	2.3 (2)	5 (5)	0.45[c]
Nephropathy	1.1 (1)	2 (2)	>0.99[c]
Diabetic foot	3.4 (3)	5.9 (6)	0.51[c]
Polypharmacy			0.31[a]
≥4 medications	75 (66)	82.2 (83)	
Depression symptoms by BDI score			>0.99[a]
Positive score	15.9 (14)	16 (16)	
Smoking			0.16[c]
Smoker	8 (7)	9.9 (10)	
Never smoked	58 (51)	59.4 (60)	
Former smoker	34 (30)	30.7 (31)	
Alcohol consumption			0.07[a]
Above maximum dose/week	2.3 (2)	9.9 (10)	
Time of physical exercise[e]			0.16[a]
<150 minutes/week	78.4 (69)	87.1 (88)	
≥150 minutes/week	21.6 (19)	12.9 (13)	

(continued on next page)

e208   *Steffen et al / Am J Prev Med 2021;60(5):e203−e212*

Table 1. Comparison of Baseline Sociodemographic and Health History Characteristics of Patients (*continued*)

Variables	Usual care, % (*n*) (*n*=88)	Test/MI, % (*n*) (*n*=101)	*p*-value
Regular medical follow-up for T2DM/AH			0.31[a]
Minimum of 1 consultation per year	71.3 (62)	65.3 (66)	
Consultation with a nurse in the previous year			0.02[a]
Yes	14.8 (13)	4 (4)	
No	85.2 (75)	96 (97)	
Adherence—MBG Questionnaire			0.43[c]
Total adherence	42 (37)	34.7 (35)	
Partial adherence	58 (51)	64.4 (65)	
No adherence	0.0 (0)	1 (1)	

[a]*p*-value obtained from chi-square test.
[b]Value obtained by *t*-test.
[c]Value obtained by Fisher's exact test.
[d]Minimum wage: R$998,00.
[e]Time in minutes per week.
AH, arterial hypertension; BDI, Beck Depression Inventory; CVD, cardiovascular disease; MBG, Martín−Bayarre−Grade Questionnaire; MI, motivational interviewing; T2DM, Type 2 diabetes mellitus.

it impossible to collect the final data (Figure 1). The measurement of the main outcome involved blood tests, and blood samples had to be collected in another outpatient clinic, so these were factors that led to dropouts.

Table 1 shows the characteristics of the test/MI and usual care groups. There were no significant differences between the groups for most of the baseline characteristics. An exception was the variable of consultation with the nurse in the previous year, which was statistically adjusted as described in the data analysis because it represented a higher amount of intervention received by the usual-care group from baseline. The mean age of the participants was 66 (SD=9.91) years; most had a diagnosis of T2DM and AH for >10 years and were on a polypharmacy regimen with regular medical follow-up in the previous year, had partial levels of adherence, and were nonsmokers and sedentary.

Table 2 shows the comparison between the groups for the outcomes investigated before and after the interventions. At the conclusion of the study, there were no statistically significant differences in HbA1c levels (*p*=0.07) between the groups. However, at the end of the study, there was a 0.4% (*p*<0.01) reduction in HbA1c levels for the test/MI group with a statistical significance and a small effect size (0.3). There was no significant difference in HbA1c levels of the participants in the usual-care group (−0.1%, *p*=0.70).

There were statistically significant differences between groups with improvement in the test/MI group for the outcomes SBP (*p*<0.01), diastolic BP (DBP) (*p*<0.01), total Martín−Bayarre−Grade adherence score (*p*=0.04), and Martín−Bayarre−Grade questionnaire dimensions of treatment adherence and personal involvement (*p*=0.03 and *p*=0.04). The test/MI group had a significant

mean reduction of 13.7 mmHg in SBP compared with the usual-care group, with a large effect size (0.87). Regarding DBP, there was a decrease of 5.7 mm Hg with a medium effect size (0.71). For adherence, the magnitude of the effect found was reduced (0.29).

As a secondary outcome, nurses referred patients to a general practitioner for a review consultation, depending on the identified needs, in 60.7% (*n*=51) of the usual-care group participants and 69.7% (*n*=69) of the test/MI group (*p*=0.26). Moreover, 31 (30.7%) participants in the test/MI group and 16 (18.2%) in the usual-care group required therapeutic maintenance until the conclusion of the study, with increased or reduced doses of drugs such as antihypertensives, antidiabetics, antidyslipidemic drugs, and antidepressants. In this regard, there was no difference between the groups (*p*=0.07).

DISCUSSION

This trial compared nursing consultations on the basis of MI with usual care nursing visits in 174 participants with T2DM and AH. It found differences between the groups with improvements in the test/MI group for BP and adherence score after a mean follow-up of 6 months. The 0.4% reduction in HbA1c levels (*p*<0.01) among participants who received MI was clinically relevant, especially considering that MI was used as an adjunct and part of the care routine for diabetes management in primary health care.[7,34] However, MI was no more effective than the usual care in reducing HbA1c levels. Mean baseline HbA1c levels of participants, associated with other characteristics such as age, time of diagnosis, polypharmacy, and associated diseases, may have represented a restricted margin for reduction according to the

Steffen et al / Am J Prev Med 2021;60(5):e203−e212   e209

Table 2. Comparison of Intragroup Results and Between Test/MI and Usual Care Groups at Baseline and at Study Completion

Variables	n	Baseline Mean ± SD	p-value Baseline[a]	Study completion Mean ± SD	Delta value Intragroup Mean (95% CI)	p-value Intragroup[b]	Effect size (Cohen's d) (95% CI)	Adjusted delta value between groups Mean (95% CI)	p-value Between groups	Adjusted difference between groups Mean (95% CI)[c]
Clinical outcomes										
HbA1c, %			0.82						0.07	
Test/MI	101	7.6 ± 1.6		7.2 ± 1.4	−0.4 (−0.7, −0.2)	**<0.01**	0.31	−0.4 (−0.7, −0.1)		−0.3 (−0.6, 0)
Usual care	88	7.5 ± 1.6		7.5 ± 1.7	−0.1 (−0.3, 0.2)	0.60		−0.1 (−0.4, 0.1)		
SBP (mm Hg)			**0.03**						**<0.01**	
Test/MI	101	147.2 ± 23.3		132.7 ± 18.4	−14.4 (−18, −10.8)	**<0.01**	0.87	−13.5 (−18.5, −8.6)		−13.7 (−18.5, −8.9)
Usual care	88	139.9 ± 21		142.3 ± 20.3	+2.4 (−1.7, 6.6)	0.26		+0.21 (−4.4, 4.8)		
DBP (mm Hg)			0.30						**<0.01**	
Test/MI	101	75.1 ± 10.7		68.7 ± 9.8	−6.4 (−8.2, −4.7)	**<0.01**	0.71	−5.4 (−8, −2.8)		−5.7 (−8.2, −3.2)
Usual care	88	73.5 ± 11		67.8 ± 9.4	0.3 (−1.7, 2.3)	0.77		+0.3 (−2.2, 2.8)		
Self-administered questionnaires										
Total MBG adherence score			0.43						**0.04**	
Test/MI	101	34.3 ± 7.3		38.4 ± 5.9	4.1 (2.9, 5.4)	**<0.01**	0.29	+4.6 (3, 6.1)		+1.5 (0.1, 3)
Usual care	88	35.1 ± 6.2		37.4 ± 5.7	2.3 (1.1, 3.4)	**<0.01**		+3 (1.6, 4.5)		
MBG score by dimensions										
Treatment adherence			0.42						**0.03**	
Test/MI	101	13.5 ± 2.2		14.3 ± 1.6	0.8 (0.4, 1.2)	**<0.01**	0.32	+1 (0.3, 1.1)		+0.5 (0, 1)
Usual care	88	13.8 ± 1.6		14 ± 1.7	0.2 (−0.1, 0.5)	0.19		+0.3 (−0.2, 0.7)		
Personal implication			0.27						**0.04**	
Test/MI	101	13.6 ± 3.2		14.7 ± 3.1	1.1 (0.5, 1.7)	**<0.01**	0.13	+2.1 (0.9, 3.3)		+1 (0, 1.6)
Usual care	88	13.1 ± 3.2		13.8 ± 31.3	0.7 (0.04, 1.4)	**0.04**		+1.2 (−0.1, 2.4)		
Therapist–patient relationship			0.06						0.56	
Test/MI	101	7.2 ± 4.1		9.6 ± 3	2.4 (1.6, 3.1)	**<0.01**	0.26	+2.2 (1.4, 3)		+0.2 (−0.6, 1.1)
Usual care	88	8.2 ± 3.7		9.7 ± 3	1.4 (0.7, 2.2)	**<0.01**		+2 (1.2, 2.8)		

Note: Boldface indicates statistical significance ($p<0.05$).
[a] p-value obtained by the t-test analysis.
[b] p-value obtained by GEE.
[c] p-value obtained by ANCOVA test.
DBP, diastolic blood pressure; GEE, generalized estimating equation; MBG, Martin−Bayarre−Grade Questionnaire; MI, motivational interviewing; SBP, systolic blood pressure.

clinical recommendations to individualized HbA1c goals.[7] Similar results were shown in studies that investigated MI in primary care environments on the basis of different modalities of delivery and with weak quality of evidence.[34,35]

In contrast, the significant finding of a reduction in BP levels found in favor of the test/MI group deserves to be emphasized. The differences of −13.7 mmHg (95% CI= −18.5, −8.9) in SBP and −5.7 mmHg in DBP (95% CI= −8.2, −3.2) in relation to those in the usual-care group were greater than what was found in the literature consulted. In a systematic review analyzing the effectiveness of MI in primary care, the mean effect size was also higher in BP results.[12] Ma and colleagues[36] reported lower levels of SBP and DBP in the group with MI than in the control group, with differences of 4.92 and 2.58 mmHg, respectively. In a meta-analysis of RCTs evaluating the effect of MI on BP, a significant effect was found for SBP (−1.64 mm Hg) but not for DBP (−0.58 mm Hg).[37] Although the mean baseline BP was higher in the test/MI group than in the usual-care group, the statistical adjustments, including changes in medical prescription during the period as a possible confounder, confirm that the results found were independent of these variables.

Likewise, MI was more effective than usual care in improving adherence levels among participants. The main effects of adherence in the test/MI group were seen in the domains of treatment adherence (which includes correct intake of prescribed drugs, a healthy diet, physical activity, and regular follow-up at the Health Unit) and personal involvement (which includes participation in a support network, mobilization of efforts, and the extent to which treatment decisions are shared with the patient). This suggests how much the quality of the relationship, the form of communication, and shared decision making provided by MI could be the decisive factors for the effectiveness of care.[7,16] Over the years, MI has been associated with comparable evidence of behavioral changes, such as improvement in regular medication use, cessation of substance abuse, change in eating habits, and maintenance of body weight, as well as qualitative perceptions of the patient's active role and partnership with the health professional.[9,14,15,19,21,35,36,38−42] These results corroborate those of trials that show MI as a promising strategy for the management of chronic conditions, especially regarding lifestyle interventions.[7,9−12,19,38−40]

Ultimately, the interventions in the usual-care group did not result in statistically significant improvements in intragroup clinical results or in relation to interventions in the test/MI group. These findings propose a link with the criticisms established >2 decades ago regarding the need for effective change in the current biomedical health model toward a model more centered on the patient and on the multiprofessional team.[7,16,40−43] The generalized lack of nursing follow-up for people with T2DM and AH at baseline is a cause for concern, given that the team approach is strongly recommended.[7,43] In this perspective, the effect of referral to the general practitioner and changes in medical prescription during the study period are interpreted as a positive effect of the nursing consultations because nurses play a key role in coordinating care and identifying risk factors for adherence and their repercussions for treatment.[6,7] Gabbay et al.[38] report the same findings, with nurses prompting physicians to re-evaluate the patient's medications. However, physicians did not always respond, which implies that strategies are required to reduce clinical inertia and promote interdisciplinary care.

Limitations

The main limitation of this study was that no feedback on MI was offered to nurses during the study (only before and after the 20 hours of training) to use MI in clinical practice. This impairs the analysis in terms of fidelity to the MI methods used during the interventions, and better outcomes could be achieved by professionals with higher levels of training and experience.[9,19,22]

Furthermore, the ideal sample size was not reached because of the lack of resources for the research. The existence of dropouts and the need to use the last observation carried forward for data analysis may have, together with the other limitations, generated underfit in the estimation of the parameter and reduced the effect of the intervention. In this context, the method used for the sample calculation, with the absence of a pilot study and the inclusion of all participants regardless of whether their baseline HbA1c levels were within the therapeutic target, contributed to the prediction of the restricted margin for reduction, considering the baseline profile of the study population. Finally, because this is a pragmatic trial evaluating aspects related to the follow-up of people with chronic diseases in primary care environments, with all their subjectivity, external interference, and psychosocial specificities, data allow for only a partial portrait of this population rather than an absolute one.

CONCLUSIONS

In the context of primary health care, the nursing consultation based on MI was shown to be a more effective care strategy than the usual care to improve BP levels and adherence levels in individuals with T2DM and AH. Moreover, MI was demonstrated to be useful in reducing HbA1c levels in diabetes management, even in a short

Steffen et al / Am J Prev Med 2021;60(5):e203−e212

e211

time. Therefore, it is hoped that this study will contribute to the consolidation of MI as an effective tool for improving care responses in chronic conditions. Nevertheless, additional evidence is needed to examine and support the forms of implementation of MI in primary care with larger and more representative samples for evaluating the effects on the professional skills and on the knowledge, attitudes, and outcomes of patients with T2DM, particularly in HbA1c levels.[14,34,35,44]

Finally, qualitative scientific methodologies should be included to determine how people receiving treatment for hypertension and diabetes who receive MI and the professionals who apply MI feel about it, which can be another good reason to implement MI widely in primary care settings, aiming to transform the healthcare reality, raise standards, and promote lifestyle changes.

ACKNOWLEDGMENTS

No financial disclosures were reported by the authors of this paper.

REFERENCES

1. WHO. *World Health Statistics 2018: Monitoring Health for the SDGs, Sustainable Development Goals.* Geneva, Switzerland: WHO, 2018.
2. Felipe GF, de Abreu RN, Moreira TM. Aspects of the nursing appointments with hypertensive patients cared for in the Family Health Program [in Portuguese]. *Rev Esc Enferm USP.* 2008;42(4):620−627. https://doi.org/10.1590/s0080-62342008000400002.
3. Glynn LG, Murphy AW, Smith SM, Schroeder K, Fahey T. Interventions used to improve control of blood pressure in patients with hypertension. *Cochrane Database Syst Rev.* 2010(3):CD005182. https://doi.org/10.1002/14651858.cd005182.pub4.
4. Welch G, Garb J, Zagarins S, Lendel I, Gabbay RA. Nurse diabetes case management interventions and blood glucose control: results of a meta-analysis. *Diabetes Res Clin Pract.* 2010;88(1):1−6. https://doi.org/10.1016/j.diabres.2009.12.026.
5. Moura Dde J, Bezerra ST, Moreira TM, Fialho AV. Nursing care to the client with hypertension: a bibliographic review. *Rev Bras Enferm.* 2011;64(4):759−765. https://doi.org/10.1590/s0034-71672011000400020.
6. WHO. Enhancing nursing and midwifery capacity to contribute to the prevention, treatment and management of noncommunicable diseases. Geneva, Switzerland: WHO. https://www.who.int/hrh/resources/observer12/en/. Published 2013. Accessed June 11, 2019.
7. American Diabetes Association. Introduction: standards of medical care in diabetes - 2020. *Diabetes Care.* 2020;43(suppl 1):S1−S2. https://doi.org/10.2337/dc20-sint.
8. Brasil, Ministério da Saúde, Secretaria de Ciência, Tecnologia e Insumos Estratégicos, Departamento de Ciência e Tecnologia. Síntese de evidências para políticas de saúde: adesão ao tratamento medicamentoso por pacientes portadores de doenças crônicas. Brasília, Brasil: Ministério da Saúde. https://pesquisa.bvsalud.org/portal/resource/pt/biblio-971867. Published 2016. Accessed August 23, 2019.
9. Steinberg MP, Miller WR. Motivational Interviewing in Diabetes Care (Applications of Motivational Interviewing). New York, NY: Guilford Press, 2015. https://doi.org/10.7861/clinmedicine.16-2-205.
10. Lundahl BW, Burke BL. The effectiveness and applicability of motivational interviewing: a practice-friendly review of four meta-analyses. *J Clin Psychol.* 2009;65(11):1232−1245. https://doi.org/10.1002/jclp.20638.
11. Cedillo IG, Antúnez BV. Eficacia de la entrevista motivacional para promover la adherencia terapéutica en pacientes con diabetes mellitus tipo 2. *Universitas Psychologica.* 2015;14(2):511−522. https://doi.org/10.11144/javeriana.upsy14-2.eemp.
12. Vanbuskirk KA, Wetherell JL. Motivational interviewing used in primary care populations: a systematic review and meta-analysis. *J Behav Med.* 2014;37(4):768−780. https://doi.org/10.1007/s10865-013-9527-4.
13. Andretta I, Meyer E, Kuhn RP, Rigon M. A entrevista motivacional no Brasil: uma revisão sistemática. *Mudanças − Psicologia da Saúde.* 2014;22(2):15−21. https://doi.org/10.15603/2176-1019/mud.v22n2p15-21.
14. Thepwongsa I, Muthukumarb R, Kessomboon P. Motivational interviewing by general practitioners for type 2 diabetes patients: a systematic review. *Fam Pract.* 2017;34(4):376−383. https://doi.org/10.1093/fampra/cmx045.
15. Dellasega C, Añel-Tiangco RM, Gabbay RA. How patients with type 2 diabetes mellitus respond to motivational interviewing. *Diabetes Res Clin Pract.* 2012;95(1):37−41. https://doi.org/10.1016/j.diabres.2011.08.011.
16. Dickinson JK, Guzman SJ, Maryniuk MD, et al. The use of language in diabetes care and education. *Diabetes Care.* 2017;40(12):1790−1799. https://doi.org/10.2337/dci17-0041.
17. Mendes EV. O cuidado das condições crônicas na atenção primária à saúde: o imperativo da consolidação da estratégia da saúde da família. Brasília, Brasil: Organização Pan-Americana da Saúde. http://bvsms.saude.gov.br/bvs/publicacoes/cuidado_condicoes_atencao_primaria_saude.pdf. Published 2012. Accessed July 15, 2019.
18. Centro Colaborador da OMS para a Classificação de Doenças em Português-CBCD. Classificação Estatística Internacional de Doenças e Problemas relacionados à Saúde-10ª. Revisão. São Paulo, Brasil: Centro Latino-Americano e do Caribe de Informação em Ciências da Saúde. https://pesquisa.bvsalud.org/portal/resource/pt/lis-LISBR1.1-16207. Published 2001. Accessed July 15, 2019.
19. Chen SM, Creedy D, Lin HS, Wollin J. Effects of motivational interviewing intervention on self-management, psychological and glycemic outcomes in type 2 diabetes: a randomized controlled trial. *Int J Nurs Stud.* 2012;49(6):637−644. https://doi.org/10.1016/j.ijnurstu.2011.11.011.
20. Brasil, Ministério da Saúde, Grupo Hospitalar Conceição, Gerência de Saúde Comunitária. A organização do cuidado às pessoas com hipertensão arterial sistêmica em serviços de atenção primária à saúde. Organização de Sandra R. S. Ferreira, Itemar M. Bianchini, Rui Flores. Porto Alegre, Brasil: Hospital Nossa Senhora daConceição. https://ensinoepesquisa.ghc.com.br/images/Publicacao/a%20organizao%20do%20cuidado.pdf. Published 2011. Accessed August 18, 2019.
21. Miller WR, Rollnick S. *Motivational Interviewing: Helping People Change.* 3rd ed. New York, NY: Guilford Press, 2013.
22. Moyers TB, Martin T, Manuel JK, Miller WR, Ernst D. *Revised global scales: Motivational Interviewing Treatment Integrity 3.0 (MITI 3.0).* Albuquerque, NM: University of New Mexico, Center on Alcoholism, Substance Abuse and Addictions (CASAA); 2007. https://casaa.unm.edu/download/miti3.pdf.
23. Miller WR, Hedrick KE, Orlofsky DR. The Helpful Responses Questionnaire: a procedure for measuring therapeutic empathy. *J Clin Psychol.* 1991;47(3):444−448. https://doi.org/10.1002/1097-4679(199105)47:3≤444::aid-jclp2270470320≥3.0.co;2-u.
24. Miller WR, Moyers TB, Ernst D, Amrhein P. *Manual for the Motivational Interviewing Skill Code (MISC) Version 2.1.* Albuquerque, NM: University of New Mexico, Center on Alcoholism, Substance Abuse and Addictions; 2008. http://casaa.unm.edu/download/misc.pdf.
25. Lord SP, Can D, Yi M, et al. Advancing methods for reliably assessing motivational interviewing fidelity using the motivational interviewing skills code. *J Subst Abuse Treat.* 2015;49:50−57. https://doi.org/10.1016/j.jsat.2014.08.005.
26. Nerenberg KA, Zarnke KB, Leung AA, et al. Hypertension Canada's 2018 Guidelines for Diagnosis, Risk Assessment, Prevention, and Treatment of Hypertension in Adults and Children. *Can J Cardiol.* 2018;34(5):506−525. https://doi.org/10.1016/j.cjca.2018.02.022.

27. Huang Y, Wei X, Wu T, Chen R, Guo A. Collaborative care for patients with depression and diabetes mellitus: a systematic review and meta-analysis. *BMC Psychiatry.* 2013;13(1):260. https://doi.org/10.1186/1471-244x-13-260.

28. Gorestein C, Andrade L. Inventário de depressão de Beck: propriedades psicométricas da versão em português. *Rev Psiq Clín.* 1998;25(5):245–250. http://bases.bireme.br/cgi-bin/wxislind.exe/iah/online/?IsisScript=iah/iah.xis&src=google&base=LILACS&lang=p&nextAction=lnk&exprSearch=228051&indexSearch=ID. Accessed February 10, 2021.

29. Cunha JA. *Manual da versão em português das Escalas Beck.* São Paulo, SP: Casa do Psicólogo, 2001.

30. Matta R, Luiza S, Lucia V, Azeredo TB. Adaptação brasileira de questionário para avaliar adesão terapêutica em hipertensão arterial. *Rev Saúde Pública.* 2013;47(2):292–300. https://doi.org/10.1590/s0034-8910.2013047003463.

31. Alfonso LM, Vea HDB, Ábalo JA. Validación del cuestionario MBG (Martín-Bayarre-Grau) para evaluar la adherencia terapéutica en hipertensión arterial. *Rev Cub Salud Pública.* 2008;34(1).. https://doi.org/10.1590/s0864-34662008000100012.

32. WHO. Adherence to Long Term Therapies: Evidence for Action. Geneva, Switzerland: WHO, 2003.

33. Resolução Cofen n° 0544/2017. Cofen. http://www.cofen.gov.br/resolucao-cofen-no-05442017_52029.html. Updated May 18, 2017. Accessed May 12, 2017.

34. Christie D, Channon S. The potential for motivational interviewing to improve outcomes in the management of diabetes and obesity in paediatric and adult populations: a clinical review. *Diabetes Obes Metab.* 2014;16(5):381–387. https://doi.org/10.1111/dom.12195.

35. Ekong G, Kavookjian J. Motivational interviewing and outcomes in adults with type 2 diabetes: a systematic review. *Patient Educ Couns.* 2015;99(6):944–952. https://doi.org/10.1016/j.pec.2015.11.022.

36. Ma C, Zhou Y, Zhou W, Huang C. Evaluation of the effect of motivational interviewing counselling on hypertension care. *Patient Educ Couns.* 2014;95(2):231–237. https://doi.org/10.1016/j.pec.2014.01.011.

37. Ren Y, Yang H, Browning C, Thomas S, Liu M. Therapeutic effects of motivational interviewing on blood pressure control: a meta-analysis of randomized controlled trials. *Int J Cardiol.* 2014;172(2):509–511. https://doi.org/10.1016/j.ijcard.2014.01.051.

38. Gabbay RA, Añel-Tiangco RM, Dellasega C, Mauger DT, Adelman A, Van Horn DHA. Diabetes nurse case management and motivational interviewing for change (DYNAMIC): results of a 2-year randomized controlled pragmatic trial. *J Diabetes.* 2013;5(3):349–357. https://doi.org/10.1111/1753-0407.12030.

39. Martins RK, McNeil DW. Review of motivational interviewing in promoting health behaviors. *Clin Psychol Rev.* 2009;29(4):283–293. https://doi.org/10.1016/j.cpr.2009.02.001.

40. Song D, Xu TZ, Sun QH. Effect of motivational interviewing on self-management in patients with type 2 diabetes mellitus: a meta-analysis. *Int J Nurs Sci.* 2014;1(3):291–297. https://doi.org/10.1016/j.ijnss.2014.06.002.

41. Fisher L, Polonsky WH, Hessler D, Potter MB. A practical framework for encouraging and supporting positive behaviour change in diabetes. *Diabet Med.* 2017;34(12):1658–1666. https://doi.org/10.1111/dme.13414.

42. Rutten GEHM, Alzaid A. Person-centred type 2 diabetes care: time for a paradigm shift. *Lancet Diabetes Endocrinol.* 2018;6(4):264–266. https://doi.org/10.1016/s2213-8587(17)30193-6.

43. Williams B, Mancia G, Spiering W, Rosei EA, Azizi M, Burnier M. 2019 ESC Guidelines on diabetes, pre-diabetes, and cardiovascular diseases developed in collaboration with the EASD: the Task Force for diabetes, pre-diabetes, and cardiovascular diseases of the European Society of Cardiology (ESC) and the European Association for the Study of Diabetes (EASD). *Eur Heart J.* 2018;34(39):3021–3104. https://doi.org/10.1093/eurheartj/eht108.

44. Jansink R, Braspenning J, Keizer E, van der Weijden T, Elwyn G, Grol R. No identifiable Hb1Ac or lifestyle change after a comprehensive diabetes programme including motivational interviewing: a cluster randomised trial. *Scand J Prim Health Care.* 2013;31(2):119–127. https://doi.org/10.3109/02813432.2013.797178.

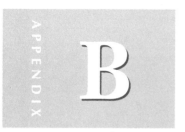

Qualitative Study

Applied Nursing Research 57 (2021) 151390

Contents lists available at ScienceDirect

Applied Nursing Research

journal homepage: www.elsevier.com/locate/apnr

A grounded theory approach to the care experience of patients with intravenous drug use/abuse-related endocarditis ☆

Jennifer P. Colwill, DNP, APRN-CNS, CCNS, PCCN, Clinical Nurse Specialist [a, *],
Minerva I. Sherman, MSN, APRN, ACNP, Certified Nurse Practitioner [b], Sandra L. Siedlecki, PhD,
RN, APRN, FAAN, Senior Nurse Scientist [c], Christian N. Burchill, PhD, MSN, RN, CEN, Director
of Nursing Research and Science [d], Lee Anne Siegmund, PhD, RN, ACSM-CEP, Nurse Scientist II [c]

[a] Nursing Institute
[b] Heart Vascular and Thoracic Institute, Cardiothoracic Department, Cleveland Clinic, Cleveland, OH, United States of America
[c] Office of Nursing Research and Innovation, Cleveland Clinic, Cleveland, OH, United States of America
[d] Penn Medicine, Lancaster General Health, Lancaster, Pennsylvania, USA

1. Introduction

Hospital admissions for person(s) who inject drugs (PWID) with infective endocarditis have doubled over the last decade(Kadri et al., 2019; Weiss et al., 2020), and surgical intervention is needed to improve survival (Long & Koyfman, 2018). PWID with infective endocarditis (hereafter referred to as endocarditis) have poorer surgical outcomes (Hussain et al., 2017; Kim et al., 2016; Rabkin et al., 2012; Rudasill et al., 2019; Shrestha et al., 2015; Silaschi et al., 2017) including need for reoperation due to post-surgical relapse. This often creates ethical dilemmas for providers (DiMaio et al., 2009; Hull & Jadbabaie, 2014). Some healthcare workers in the U.S. and abroad hold negative stereotypes of PWID, adversely affecting access to needed services (Guise et al., 2016; Ibragimov et al., 2017; Kennedy-Hendricks et al., 2016; Klingemann, 2017; Lang et al., 2013; Pollini, 2017). Individuals perceive these negative stereotypes from healthcare workers as feelings of humiliation and lack of fairness and dignity in healthcare settings (Klingemann, 2017). This creates a situation in which PWID feel the need to hide their addiction from providers, further resulting in reduced access to care (Biancarelli et al., 2019). In a study that explored perception of care in both the inpatient and outpatient settings, researchers found that PWID with endocarditis identified stigma, physical and social co-morbidities, an expected return to abuse, and lack of care coordination as common experiences when interacting with the healthcare system (Bearnot et al., 2019). Researchers have not exclusively explored the hospitalized patient perspective in this unique population of PWID with endocarditis as they await a treatment decision. We sought to address the gap in the literature, recognizing that these patients are a rich resource regarding their own complex needs.

2. Methods

The research question for this study was: *How do PWID hospitalized with endocarditis interpret their lives as they move in and out of the hospital and society?* The aim of this study was to develop a model to describe these phenomena. A grounded theory approach with semi-structured interviews following methods described by Strauss and Corbin was used (Strauss & Corbin, 1998). Grounded theory was chosen since it is appropriate for generating and refining theories or models (Chun Tie et al., 2019). This study was approved by the hospital's Institutional Review Board and written informed consent was obtained from all participants.

2.1. Participants

This study was conducted in the inpatient setting within a quaternary care medical center in the Midwest. Inclusion criteria were adult PWID hospitalized with endocarditis undergoing evaluation for surgical management. Those who could not participate in an in-person interview conducted in English were excluded. Theoretical purposive sampling methods were used (Strauss & Corbin, 1998).

2.2. Procedures

Potential participants were identified from patient lists of those undergoing surgical evaluation for endocarditis. The electronic medical

☆ No external funding was received for this project.The authors have no conflicts of interest to disclose.
* Corresponding author at: 9500 Cleveland Clinic, Mail Box P3 112-01, Cleveland, OH 44195, United States of America.
  E-mail address: colwilj@ccf.org (J.P. Colwill).

https://doi.org/10.1016/j.apnr.2020.151390
Received 2 July 2020; Received in revised form 5 August 2020; Accepted 21 November 2020
Available online 25 November 2020
0897-1897/© 2020 Elsevier Inc. All rights reserved.

J.P. Colwill et al.

Applied Nursing Research 57 (2021) 151390

record was reviewed to identify those with a diagnosis of substance use/abuse disorder and individuals were approached for participation. Individuals were consented and an interview was scheduled. One-on-one interviews were digitally recorded and conducted in private patient rooms. Self-reported demographic characteristics were collected prior to the interview. Grand Tour questions were read from a script (Box 1). Relevant follow-up questions, based on individuals' verbal and non-verbal communication, were asked to further elucidate participants' thoughts and feelings.

Two investigators (JC and MS) conducted interviews between June and November 2019. JC is a clinical nurse specialist in cardiovascular step-down with expertise in nursing care for cardiovascular surgical patients, and a background in counseling and psychotherapy. MS is nurse practitioner specializing in care of cardiothoracic surgery patients. Additionally, three nurse scientists, LS, CB, and SS, skilled in qualitative research, participated. JC and MS were trained by LS, CB, and SS through role playing and practice prior to data collection. After each of the first few interviews LS, CB and SS listened to interview recordings and gave critical reviews of technique.

2.3. Data analysis

A member of the research team transcribed the interviews verbatim, and the team used both the audio recordings and transcripts to identify themes following the constant comparative method (Strauss & Corbin, 1998). Analysis and interviews were concurrent. Data were read and reread, and copious memos written and reviewed. Based on coding and interviewing processes, a final model was developed. Model development included a total of 20 iterations, including reviewing the data and redrawing the model. Relevant content was categorized and given meaning (open coding) (Strauss & Corbin, 1998). Relationships between categorized themes were identified (axial coding) (Strauss & Corbin, 1998). The interconnections of the themes required a process of identifying the meaning that the individuals ascribed to the events of their lives, consistent with 'evolved' grounded theory, in which symbolic meaning is given to social interactions (Chun Tie et al., 2019; Strauss & Corbin, 1998). Axial coding also included constant comparison and memoing to confirm that the themes fit the emerging model. Finally, codes were selectively tied together, resulting in a core concept and articulation of a final model (selective coding) (Strauss & Corbin, 1998).

Theoretical saturation was reached when, concepts of the emerging model with no new themes surfaced and, the team developed a good understanding of the recurring themes (Sbaraini et al., 2011). Discrepancies were resolved through iterations, numerous discussions, and going back to the data. This included using dialogue to resolve appropriate terminology when referencing the individuals, their disease processes, and core concepts. Once the team agreed that saturation had been reached, 3 additional interviews were conducted.

3. Results

Eleven participants (hereafter referred to as individuals) were interviewed over a period of one year. The sample was female (5),

Caucasian (7), married (3), and employed (3). Interviews ranged from 7 to 31 min and were driven by the individual (Table 1). Pseudonyms are used in order to maintain participant confidentiality and anonymity. A model for PWID hospitalized with endocarditis was developed from the analyzed data.

3.1. The model

The model presented here is the integration of categories that emerged from the data and describes the core concept of cyclical life experiences of PWID who are hospitalized with endocarditis (Fig. 1). The model is made up of 2 inter-related cycles we called *The Person* and *The Healthcare System*, that exist within the cycle of *Society*. Endocarditis is the catalyst that initiates change and drives the process forward as the individual enters *The Healthcare System*. Expressions of hope and hopelessness co-exist with behaviors of the use/abuse cycle still present whether the individual was in *The Healthcare System* or *Society*. Quotations by the individuals are used to explicate the model.

3.2. Major themes

3.2.1. The person

The Person cycle represents cyclical experiences and processes of being a PWID. *The Person* cycle describes the loss of who they had been; their sense of self-identity was now being defined by their drug use with an ongoing struggle to reclaim that lost identity.

> Phil: (Crying) *I have nothing but regret. I turned into a person that I don't know. This is not who I am."*

At the same time, they wanted others to see them as a person, not as an *"addict"* or a *"junkie"*. Desperation and ongoing drug use was part of that cycle.

> Matt: *"I don't know why I decided to screw it up for 15 years with drugs and I feel horrible. I went to prison…and I still decided to keep using."*

The following sub-themes were identified: Want to die, Loss of control, and Withdrawal.

3.2.1.1. Want to die.
Want to die represents a fixation on dying while using/abusing injectable drugs. Some expressed thoughts about wanting to die or that death was better than life. Death was very much a part of their lives.

> Sarah: *"So many times I wanted to go somewhere and curl up in a ball and die and…when you do 'like heroin' [you] feel like you don't really care… at that point you don't care if you die or not. There were times that we (discussing her relationship with her boyfriend who is also injects drugs) wanted that (referring to dying) and we'd do too much [drugs] and go to sleep holding each other and it just didn't happen for us."*

> Matt: *"Death may be a good thing for me at this point in my life; there will be peace and relaxation…the only sadness I feel is for my family 'cause I*

Box 1
. Grand tour questions.

a. Tell me what it is like being admitted to the hospital.
b. Follow-up questions included:
   i. Tell me more about _____ .
   ii. You mentioned _____ can you go into more detail about _____ ?
   iii. I would like to hear more about _____ .
   iv. You mentioned _____ tell me how that made you feel.

J.P. Colwill et al.

Applied Nursing Research 57 (2021) 151390

Table 1
Characteristics of persons who inject drugs hospitalized with endocarditis.

Pseudonym	Sex	Age (years)	Marital status	Education	Race	Employment	Household income $ (annual)	Place of residence
Sarah	F	25	Divorced	HS	C	UE	<50 K	With family
Matt	M	32	Single	HS	C	UE	50-100 K	Homeless
Ellen	F	40	Single	Above HS	C	E	<50 K	With family
Tanya	F	32	NR	NR	NR	NR	NR	NR
Samuel	M	39	Married	Other	C	D	NR	On my own
Brenda	F	NR	NR	NR	C	NR	NR	NR
Patrick	M	29	Single	HS	NC	UE	NR	With family
Carlos	M	24	Divorced	HS	C	E	<50 K	With family
John	M	30	Married	Less than HS	Other	E	<50 K	With a friend
Phil	M	29	Married	Less than HS	C	UE	NR	With a friend
Marie	F	NR	NR	NR	NR	NR	NR	NR

M, male; F, female; NR, not reported; HS, high school; C, Caucasian; NC, non-Caucasian; E, employed; UE, unemployed; D, disability; K, $1000.

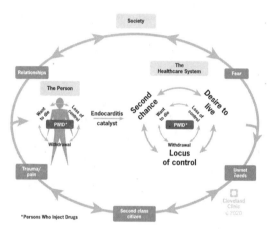

Fig. 1. PWID with Endocarditis Cyclical Experiences (PEaCE) model.

know they will be upset. I know I will be at peace once I am dead just because of the life I've been living.

John: *"Don't let no one talk you into it...they're trying to kill you* (referring to other drug users). *If people cared about you they would at least call* (talking about being in the hospital). *They don't care about me...I'm on my death bed."*

3.2.1.2. Loss of control. Individuals reported a loss of control to their addiction as Carlos described, *"You are always chasing that high."* Individuals viewed their lives as being a never ending ritual of substance use. They no longer recalled the ritual's purpose; they felt no control over their ritualistic behavior.

Sarah: *"Being on heroin is like living on a roller coaster. I didn't like who I was anymore. I was upset and mad and didn't know what to do. ....not only was I addicted to the drug, but I was addicted to the ritual of doing it. I have to do it after I eat, I have to do it after this and this...and it's constant and every day. You're on a constant chase; it consumes your life".*

Phil: *"It spirals out of control and it won't let go of you till something bad happens. Every time something bad happens it always kills me and still for some dumb reason I keep going down that path and I don't want to go down that path* (starts crying)... *no more".*

3.2.1.3. Withdrawal. Withdrawal was described as a negative experience to be avoided at all cost. For many, anything was better than the

dreadful sickness of withdrawal, including the decision to keep using drugs.

Sarah: *"At first you get high and you feel good. Then you almost never get high...you just want to be Un-sick. Being sick is completely miserable".*

Matt: *"You quit doing drugs and you feel like you are going to die".*

Tanya: *"It makes you sick if you take it and makes you sick if you don't take it".*

3.2.2. The healthcare system

Endocarditis was the reason the individuals were in the *Healthcare System.* A number of them talked about endocarditis as the defining moment for them, a catalyst that kindled their recognition of a need to change. It was a pause that gave them a chance to reevaluate their lives. Although they expressed that they knew the healthcare system was there to help, they didn't always feel supported in their desire to live or end their addiction.

Samuel: *"I feel like the system is broken and it collapsed on top of me."*

Tanya: *"You are not even worthy for them to talk to you or worth their time...right now it feels like a death sentence. Like nobody wants to work on me or help me."*

At the same time the individuals felt they had no control over decisions providers made about their lives. They felt a desire to regain the control over their lives they lost to their addiction. The following subthemes were identified: second chance, desire to live, and locus of control.

3.2.2.1. Second chance. Individuals described feeling that contracting endocarditis actually gave them a second chance at a better life. The hospitalization that resulted from endocarditis, and fear of the diagnosis, became an opportunity to look at their lives and refocus on the people and things that really mattered to them. For some, this was punctuated by a sense of determination and even optimism.

Patrick: *"I do not want to do drugs. It was a second chance at life. They told me I would not last 10 hours. When they told me that, it changed my whole state on life and drugs itself."*

John: *"I was in the county jail and I guess I had a temp of 107 degrees, and they called the paramedics. That's the worst I ever imagined [could happen] from doing heroin. I don't ever want to do drugs again. I don't know how my life is going to change. I just know it is. No more drugs. I might be able to tell you a story down the road when I'm clean...I've never been clean."*

Marie: *"I got a second chance. Like my brother said, you only get so many chances. I'm going to my brother's and do rehab and I'm going to make it."*

3

J.P. Colwill et al.

Applied Nursing Research 57 (2021) 151390

3.2.2.2. Desire to live. For those that saw endocarditis as a growth opportunity and even for some of those who didn't, there was an expressed desire to live, to choose life over addiction. Some individuals were in the evaluation process awaiting a decision on surgery as an option, and others had already received word that they were not surgical candidates. For the subset of the population who were not surgical candidates, they still had a strong desire to live but knew they would most likely die due to complications from endocarditis.

> Matt: *"Now I just want to live; it is so important to me to stay alive and I don't care if I don't have to do drugs again ever in my life and I say that straight from the heart. So hopefully, hopefully they decided I am worth living, do this surgery and I can go into treatment; sober living after this… that is my goal just to stay alive."*

> Brenda: *"Staying sober means life to me. It is being me, the 'me' I am supposed to be."*

> Samuel: *"I was fighting for another chance to live, to provide for my family and I do not get that opportunity no more. I just get to go crawl to hospice and die and that is what my family deserves."*

3.2.2.3. Locus of control. The years of giving over decision-making control to their addiction are now replaced by giving control to caregivers in the healthcare system. Most individuals expressed resentment that providers and others made decisions for them. During their active addiction they felt a loss of control to their addiction, trapped in ritualistic behavior without decision-making authority. Now, the locus of control shifted from a loss of control over drug use/abuse to a perception that healthcare providers were now in control and sometimes ignored or minimized their wants or needs.

> Brenda: *"The whole reason I was brought [here], was because I was told that this is the one hospital willing to operate on me. Being that this is my 'second offence' if you were. And here I talked to the surgeon and he pretty much told me that he will not operate."*

> Matt: *"We are going to have to do open heart surgery on you BUT… we might not… we have to decide if my life is worth living and that is just sad that people can do that."*

> Marie: *"Being in here [in the hospital] I want to take advantage of everything. I can't go back to where I live…they always say you got to change your people, places and things and I was like 'I got this' …and I didn't have it."*

3.2.3. Society

Many individuals spoke of the norms and values in which they were raised and currently resided, and their experiences within that culture. The individuals' social circle and family influenced the way they saw drug use. Experiences became patterns of behavior that supported substance use and abuse. Many were exposed to drug use and abuse from a very young age, resulting in physical, psychological, and emotional trauma, and leading to an ongoing pattern of ineffective coping and substance use.

> Sarah: *"I come from three generations of drug use. My brother-in-law passed away from a drug overdose, my mom uses, she still uses. I've used with my mom, so that doesn't help. My mom's, like, shot me up before so that's not normal. Growing up, drugs were like a normal thing in my life."*

Some individuals expressed trepidation about leaving the hospital to go back to the same social system that helped them maintain their substance use/abuse cycle. The following sub-themes were identified: relationships, trauma and pain, second class citizens, fear, and unmet needs.

3.2.3.1. Relationships. Unhealthy relationships and poor role models often led to ineffective coping that resulted in drug use. Individuals struggled with knowing that supportive relationships are necessary to recovery and yet a desire to maintain some of the relationships from their family of origin or social circle. Some spoke to the fact that drug use and abuse has taken the life of some of their closest relations.

> Sarah: *"…and we've (discussing her relationship with her boyfriend) seen each other at our worst and we both understand the struggle. We can be there for each other. I've had a couple friends overdose and I've had to Narcan them…I can deal with their situations but others cannot. I cannot imagine a situation where I can depend on someone to Narcan me."*

> Matt: *"Well I lost… all of my friends are dead, all of my friends that use are dead… my brother overdosed and died, my father overdosed and died in front of me."*

> Ellen: *"So it was like I have such high anxiety so talking about certain things umm… I was in an abusive relationship and I could not really talk about that 'cause I did not want my kids taken away. Now it was happening behind closed doors when my kids were asleep and stuff, that was my way of numbing my pain and not talking about it because I did not want people to know what was going on."*
> *"You just really want it, you really want it (referring to being drug free). And [you need to] have good family support system."*

> Patrick: *"everyone I know who do 'do drugs' I have no connection to them and that is better (talking about moving forward)."*

3.2.3.2. Trauma and pain. Individuals identified experiences of trauma and pain as defining moments in their lives, as though they knew the exact circumstances that led to their substance use and abuse. For most the trauma and pain, whether physical, emotional, or both, became overwhelming. They described various societal influences such as growing up in families that had generational pattern of drug use/abuse, being around friends who used/abused drugs, the ease of getting legal prescription drugs that had potential for abuse, and living in neighborhoods where exposure to drug use was *"at every corner"*. The accessibility to drugs and the culture around them became an enabling environment. Meanwhile, drug use and abuse became an easy means of escape from the loneliness and pain.

> Sarah: *"It spiraled up into something….my daughter passed away. I had an IUD which perforated through my uterus and had to be cut out of my stomach…emergency surgery. I had my tubes removed. 90 Percocet's or so in a weeks' time. It was a very dark time for me…alone…[I] started using prescription, then heroin, and moved up from there."*

> Phil: *"Once you get into that same mind (referring to drug use) it is hard to get out of it. What you used to know, how you used to live, (referring to before drug use)… The fast paced life style that is all pain, you get so far into depression where nothing can help you. …depression it feels like nothing can help and you start numbing it with something here and something there and then… (talking about relapsed)".*

> Marie: *"I've never had nobody, nobody to care for me. It's always been me by myself. (voice cracking)…".*

3.2.3.3. Second class citizen. Individuals spoke of feeling like second class citizens within society and the healthcare environment. Individuals' perspectives in both realms were that of being judged and being treated as less than human because of their opioid use disorder. The healthcare system functions within society and is a reflection of societal values and norms surrounding opioid use disorder. Although individuals expected compassionate treatment, they perceived a double standard. Many expressed they felt they were treated differently than other patients because of their opioid use disorder.

4

J.P. Colwill et al.

Applied Nursing Research 57 (2021) 151390

In Society.

Sarah: *[I wish]…there is more understanding and less judgment. It just bothers me that people feel that type of way. People are judgmental… I really tried to hide that I was using."*

Matt: *"… then the ones that don't use do not want to be around you. When you're a drug addict you are worse than a dog on the street."*

Ellen:*" you'd be surprised how people treat addicts. They call them junkies. And everything else. We are not* (referring to the word junkies). *We choose to stick needles in our arm. We choose to do the drug…".*

In The Healthcare System.

Sarah: *"And my insurance doesn't really cover nice [skilled nursing facilities]. This one was just up the street…. It was so ghetto and under-staffed and the nurses suck and they don't give you your meds on time. It's just like, I am not an old person, I know what is going on…I don't really belong in a nursing home. I am 25 years old …".*

Matt: *"Once you are admitted as an IV drug user you automatically get treated like less than a human being …like an animal. It does not matter if you have good insurance, bad insurance, they try to discharge you right away, they don't give you good medical care, they scoff at you… they just treat you horrible."*

Brenda: *"And although the staff has been very good to me, I still feel like a somewhat lesser citizen…because of my opiate drug use, and the fact that nobody wants to give me medicine for my pain, like my pain means less than the suffering of others, because I hurt myself on the street."*

Phil: *"I know you can get [endocarditis] from other things…but in my case since it is because of drugs I feel judged right on the spot; they all put me in a box, nurses, hospital staff, they all put me in a box with all those other drug addicts. But I refuse to be put in a box. They label me as the same. It makes me feel angry, and less than human I guess. It makes me feel like I'm not worthy of their care."*

3.2.3.4. Fear. Individuals described fear from situations relating to society and the healthcare system. Fear was related to the consequences of addiction, but also endocarditis, as they faced the possibility of surgery, death, and fear of the unknown.

Ellen: *"I know I used [drugs] to escape or to numb myself."*
"I was diagnosed with PTSD and so I tried medications, counselling and I experienced a lot of trauma…it triggers memories, emotions like I'll panic and I go in panic mode and I tend to isolate myself and I run away."
"I shouldn't have to have valve replacement at 33. It makes, you know, it's a scary (speaking of going through surgery)."

Tanya: *"I was dependent on the hospital to help. Once they told me I have to have surgery, it got pretty real and pretty scary."*

3.2.3.5. Unmet needs. Unmet Needs were universal and reflected the pervasive themes of hope and hopelessness. The individuals were caught between wanting help and feeling abandoned. Transitions from society to healthcare and back again left them feeling alone in their struggles.

Ellen: *"That is the reason why I waited so long to go to the hospital because I have been judged so many times and looked at and plus I am pregnant and it is a scary thing. Maybe advocating for those who want to get hope but are too scared to get hope."*

Marie: *"It's so hard, I'm just all alone. And then I'm in here and I have my dog…I've had her 9 years…she's old as can be and nobody taking care of her. I've got friends feedin' her and stuff. I just miss my dog. And I got 2 babies. I got a 7 year old and a 12 year old. Right now they're with my ex-boyfriend's aunt. They been with her for a while now."*

3.2.4. Summary of findings

The model articulated in this study is the *PWID with Endocarditis Cyclical Experiences model (PEaCE)*, which is a visual representation of the core concept of cyclical life experiences. The findings of this study provide novel insight into ways in which PWID hospitalized with endocarditis ascribe symbolic meaning to the personal, healthcare and societal experiences and processes. They provided a history of opioid use disorder, despite the fact we did not ask about it. It was revealing that there was so much consistency between the interviews. Consistency has been recognized by Strauss and Corbin who noted that core concepts will tend to resurface in the data and all participants will relate to the concept (Strauss & Corbin, 1998). We found that endocarditis, which offered the individuals a chance for recovery, was a catalyst moving the individuals through the interdependent cycles. Hope and hopelessness along with perceptions of stigmatization were common threads throughout these cycles.

4. Discussion

To our knowledge, this is the first qualitative study to create a person-centered model developed from the perspectives of PWID who were hospitalized with endocarditis. We identified personal and systemic barriers that surround these patients, making them susceptible to sub-optimal care and negative outcomes. The subsequent model presents three themes, represented as cycles: *The Person, The Healthcare System, and Society*, which are interdependent and complex. Additionally, the hospitalized person within *The Healthcare System* was the same person outside of healthcare. They entered the hospital with the same coping skills, maladaptation, resources, and vulnerabilities. The experiences they described were much like two sides of the same coin but with different objects and people to direct those thoughts and feelings. The only difference was that endocarditis thrust them into a system and situation that opened the door to ponder change or maybe even entertain the notion of going back to who they used to be.

We found loss of control, withdrawal and wanting to die, were important sub-themes of *The Person cycle*. In a recent qualitative study, Bearnot et al. (2019) reported patients knew they would go back to drugs despite their best intentions, similarly reflecting the theme of loss of control. In addition, our research touched on a personal side of the individual, allowing for in-depth depictions of difficult encounters with death and withdrawal. These stories were often raw narratives of experiences that kept them in an endless cycle of drug use. Themes of death and withdrawal from the perspective of the PWID hospitalized with endocarditis are a new discovery for this patient population and unique to this study.

Endocarditis was the catalyst to move individuals into the healthcare system. Individuals described hospitalization as a second chance. This was a unique theme and in contrast to previous literature in which endocarditis was described as a motivator to change injection practices (Bearnot et al., 2019). The individuals in our study also described a desire to control their lives and responded to providers' decisions not to re-operate, as traumatic and a loss of control. They characterized their feelings as being treated like a second class citizen at a time when they were attempting to regain control of their lives. Similar to our study, previous work revealed that this same population perceived stigmatization and marginalization by healthcare workers (Bearnot et al., 2019; Bearnot & Mintton, 2020; Dion, 2019). Perceptions of inhuman treatment by healthcare workers in other settings has also been reported (Bearnot et al., 2019; Klingemann, 2017). Finally, although individuals in our study came from desperate situations that often left them wanting to die, they entered the healthcare system with hope and a desire to live. These findings are thematically different from the inevitable acceptance of going back to drugs reported in previous research (Bearnot et al., 2019).

Our model illustrates many of the factors that led to opioid use disorder as well as the processes experienced by PWID as they moved in and

5

Applied Nursing Research 57 (2021) 151390

out of the healthcare system and society. Many societal factors included in our model were descriptions of triggers, and issues of socialization and care integration that stood in the way of recovery. This is generally consistent with previous work addressing the problem of lack of care integration in this population (Bearnot & Mintton, 2020). In our study, these problems often related to transitions between hospital and society, represented in our model as unmet needs. Many individuals in our study also identified societal factors and traumatic events that were precursors to substance use even in early childhood. They recounted a picture of families or communities that normalized drug use. Relationship factors that led to drug use, or in some cases hope of recovery, are unique components of our model. Fear of the unknown, of relapse, or death were also important aspects of the model not previously described in qualitative literature in this specific population. As our model illustrates, individuals routinely reported facing stigma within larger society and the healthcare system. Stigmatization was a strong theme in a similar study of PWID who have endocarditis, in which physicians were also interviewed, showing a very different perspective on this problem (Bearnot et al., 2019).

4.1. Strengths and limitations

The rigor of this study is supported by the investigators' use of the concepts of confirmability, dependability, credibility, and transferability (Sikolia et al., 2013). Confirmability was evidenced by use of the constant comparative method in which the investigators considered previously collected data as new data were analyzed. All data were discussed in depth as a team. Dependability was assured through immediate transcription and review to ensure accuracy. The resulting themes were also reviewed by a drug addiction counselor. Investigators strived to maintain credibility through the use of a script to ensure the interviewer did not lead the individual. Additionally, the interviewers rehearsed follow-up questions throughout data collection and analysis. Individuals interviewed were from various backgrounds, contributing to transferability of the findings.

As with most qualitative research sample size was small, however, thematic saturation was reached. This research reflects the perspectives of PWID hospitalized with endocarditis, which may differ from non-hospitalized patients. This study was limited to individuals treated at one setting in one city in the Midwest and they may not represent others in other states or settings. We believe that due to the rigor of the study, the results can be transferred to and tested in other settings.

These results are novel in that this is the first study to our knowledge to generate a model to describe the person-centered perspective of PWID hospitalized with endocarditis. More research is needed to study optimal care pathways for these patients. The individuals themselves report a strong desire to be heard. This research provides a foundation for more effective interactions and therapeutic communication between healthcare providers and this population. The model presented here represents a framework from which person-centered care can be optimized for this very vulnerable population.

5. Conclusions

This model provides insight into the person-centered processes experienced by PWID hospitalized with endocarditis; the way they think and feel as they progress through healthcare and society. It is imperative for society and the healthcare system to find ways for reducing overt and covert stigma, a significant barrier to recovery, as we care for this population. These individuals are physiologically, psychologically and socially vulnerable. They have complex needs requiring comprehensive support systems before, during and after surgery. Beyond medical and surgical management, the model provided here can help to inform care.

CRediT authorship contribution statement

All authors contributed individually and collaboratively to this research study and manuscript:

JC: Conceptualization; Data curation; Formal analysis; Methodology; Resources; Investigation; Project administration; Validation; Visualization; Roles/Writing – original draft; Writing – review & editing. **MS:** Conceptualization; Data curation; Formal analysis; Methodology; Resources; Investigation; Validation; Visualization; Roles/Writing – original draft; Writing – review & editing. **LAS:** Conceptualization; Data curation; Formal analysis; Methodology; Resources; Investigation; Project administration; Validation; Visualization; Roles/Writing – original draft; Writing – review & editing; Supervision. **SS:** Conceptualization; Data curation; Formal analysis; Methodology; Resources; Project administration; Validation; Visualization; Roles/Writing– review & editing; Supervision. **CB:** Conceptualization; Data curation; Formal analysis; Methodology; Resources; Project administration; Validation; Visualization; Roles/Writing – review & editing.

Acknowledgments

The authors would like to thank Ken Kula for his artistic production of the final model. We would also like to acknowledge Kimberly Hutzel RN for her valuable input.

References

Bearnot, B., & Mintton, J. A. (2020). "You're always jumping through hoops": Journey mapping the care experiences of individuals with opioid use disorder-associated endocarditis. [published online ahead of print March 5, 2020]. *Journal of Addiction Medicine*. https://doi.org/10.1097/ADM.0000000000000648.

Bearnot, B., Mittona, J. A., Hayden, M., & Park, E. R. (2019). Experiences of care among individuals with opioid use disorder-associated endocarditis and their healthcare providers: Results from a qualitative study. *Journal of Substance Abuse Treatment, 102,* 16–22.

Biancarelli, D. L., Biello, K. B., Childs, E., et al. (2019). Strategies used by people who inject drugs to avoid stigma in healthcare settings. *Drug and Alcohol Dependence, 1* (198), 80–86. https://doi.org/10.1016/j.drugalcdep.2019.01.037.

Chun Tie, Y., Birks, M., & Francis, K. (2019). Grounded theory research: A design framework for novice researchers. *SAGE Open Med., 7.* https://doi.org/10.1177/2050312118822927, 2050312118822927. Published 2019 Jan 2.

DiMaio, J. M., Salerno, T. A., Bernstein, R., Araujo, K., Ricci, M., & Sade, R. M. (2009). Ethical obligation of surgeons to noncompliant patients: Can a surgeon refuse to operate on an intravenous drug-abusing patient with recurrent aortic valve prosthesis infection? *The Annals of Thoracic Surgery, 88*(1), 1–8.

Dion, K. (2019). Perceptions of persons who inject drugs about nursing care they have received. *Journal of Addictions Nursing, 30*(2), 101–107. https://doi.org/10.1097/JAN.0000000000000277.

Guise, A., Rhodes, T., Ndimbii, J., Ayon, S., & Nnaji, O. (2016). Access to HIV treatment and care for people who inject drugs in Kenya: A short report. *AIDS Care, 28*(12), 1595–1599.

Hull, S. C., & Jadbabaie, F. (2014). When is enough enough? The dilemma of value replacement in a recidivist intravenous drug user. *The Annals of Thoracic Surgery, 97* (5), 1486–1487.

Hussain, S. T., Witten, J., Shrestha, N. K., Blackstone, E. H., & Pettersson, G. B. (2017). Tricuspid valve endocarditis. *Annals of Cardiothoracic Surgery, 6*(3), 255–261. https://doi.org/10.21037/acs.2017.03.09.

Ibragimov, U., Cooper, H. L., Haardorfer, R., Denkel, K. L., Zule, W. A., & Wong, F. Y. (2017). Stigmatization of people who inject drugs (PWID) by pharmacists in Tajikistan: Sociocultural context and implications for a pharmacy based prevention approach. *Harm Reduction Journal, 16*(1), 64. https://doi.org/10.1186/s12954-017-0190-x.

Kadri, A. N., Wilner, B., Hernandez, A. V., et al. (2019). Geographic trends, patient characteristics, and outcomes of infective endocarditis associated with drug abuse in the United States from 2002 to 2016. *Journal of the American Heart Association.* https://doi.org/10.1161/JAHA.119.012969. e012969.

Kennedy-Hendricks, A., Busch, S. H., McGinty, E. E., et al. (2016). Primary care physicians' perspectives on the prescription opioid epidemic. *Drug and Alcohol Dependence, 1*(165), 61–70. https://doi.org/10.1016/j.drugalcdep.2016.05.010.

Kim, J. B., Ejiofor, J. I., Yammine, M., et al. (2016). Surgical outcomes of infective endocarditis among intravenous drug users. *The Journal of Thoracic and Cardiovascular Surgery, 52*(3). https://doi.org/10.1016/j.jtcvs.2016.02.072, 832–841.e1.

Klingemann, J. (2017). The rights of drug treatment patients: Experience of addiction treatment in Poland from a human rights perspective. *The International Journal on Drug Policy, 43,* 67–73.

Lang, K., Neil, J., Wright, J., Dell, C. A., Berenbaum, S., & El-Aneed, A. (2013). Qualitative investigation of barriers to accessing care by people who inject drugs in

6

J.P. Colwill et al.

Applied Nursing Research 57 (2021) 151390

Saskatoon, Canada: Perspectives of service providers. *Substance Abuse Treatment, Prevention, and Policy, 8*, 35. https://doi.org/10.1186/1747-597X-8-35.

Long, B., & Koyfman, A. (2018). Infectious endocarditis: An update for emergency clinicians. *The American Journal of Emergency Medicine, 36*(9), 1686–1692.

Pollini, R. A. (2017). Self-reported participation in voluntary nonprescription syringe sales in California's Central Valley. *Journal of the American Pharmaceutical Association, 57*(6), 677–685.

Rabkin, D. G., Mokadam, N. A., Miller, D. W., Goetz, R. R., Verrier, E. D., & Aldea, G. S. (2012). Long-term outcome for the surgical treatment of infective endocarditis with a focus on intravenous drug users. *The Annals of Thoracic Surgery, 93*, 51–58.

Rudasill, S. E., Sanaiha, Y., Mardock, A. L., et al. (2019). Clinical outcomes of infective endocarditis in injection drug users. *Journal of the American College of Cardiology, 73* (5), 559–570.

Sbaraini, A., Carter, S. M., Evans, R. W., & Blinkhorn, A. (2011). How to do a grounded theory study: A worked example of a study of dental practices. *BMC Medical Research Methodology, 11*, 128. https://doi.org/10.1186/1471-2288-11-128.

Shrestha, N. K., Jue, J., Hussain, S. T., et al. (2015). Injection drug use and outcomes after surgical intervention for infective endocarditis. *The Annals of Thoracic Surgery, 100*(3), 875–882. https://doi.org/10.1016/j.athoracsur.2015.03.019.

Sikolia, D., Biros, D., Mason, M., & Weiser, M. (2013). Trustworthiness of grounded theory methodology research in information systems. *Midwest Association of Information Sciences 2013 Proceedings. 16*.

Silaschi, M., Nicou, N., Deshpande, R., et al. (2017). Complicated infective aortic endocarditis: Comparison of different surgical strategies. *Interactive Cardiovascular and Thoracic Surgery, 25*(3), 343–349. https://doi.org/10.1093/icvts/ivx109.

Strauss, A., & Corbin, J. (1998). *Basics of qualitative research: Grounded theory procedures and techniques* (2nd ed.). Newbury Park, CA: Sage.

Weiss, A. J., Heslin, K. C., Stocks, C., & Owens, P. L. (2020). *Hospital inpatient stays related to opioid use disorder and endocarditis 2016; April 2020*. Healthcare Cost and Utilization Project (HCUP) Statistical Brief. URL: https://www.hcup-us.ahrq.gov/reports/statbriefs/sb256-Opioids-Endocarditis-Inpatient-Stays-2016.jsp. (Accessed 21 April 2020).

Mixed Methods Study

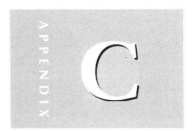

Patient Education and Counseling 104 (2021) 1222–1228

Contents lists available at ScienceDirect

Patient Education and Counseling

journal homepage: www.elsevier.com/locate/pateducou

A Mixed Methods Examination of Health Care Provider Behaviors That Build Patients' Trust

Jessica Greene[a,*], Christal Ramos[b]

[a] Marxe School of Public and International Affairs, Baruch College, City University of New York, 135 East 22nd St., Room 816D, New York, NY, 10010, USA
[b] Health Policy Center, The Urban Institute, 500 L'Enfant Plaza SW, Washington, DC, 20024, USA

ARTICLE INFO

Article history:
Received 17 April 2020
Received in revised form 3 September 2020
Accepted 5 September 2020

ABSTRACT

Objective: Patient trust in health care providers is associated with better health behaviors and utilization, yet provider trust has not been consistently conceptualized. This study uses qualitative methods to identify the key health provider behaviors that patients report build their trust, and data from a national U.S. survey of adults to test the robustness of the qualitative findings.
Methods: In this mixed methods study, we conducted 40 semi-structured interviews with a diverse sample to identify the provider behaviors that build trust. We then analyzed a nationally representative survey (n = 6,517) to examine the relationship between respondents' trust in their usual provider and the key trust-related behaviors identified in the qualitative interviews.
Results: Interviewees reported that health providers build trust by communicating effectively (listening and providing detailed explanations), caring about their patients (treating them as individuals, valuing their experience, and showing commitment to solving their health issues), and demonstrating competence (being knowledgeable, thorough, and solving their health issues). Trust in one's provider was highly correlated with all eight survey items measuring communication, caring, and competence.
Conclusions: To build trust with patients, health providers should actively listen, provide detailed explanations, show caring for patients, and demonstrate their knowledge.

© 2020 Published by Elsevier B.V.

1. Introduction

Trusting one's physician has long been considered essential for an effective patient-physician relationship [1–3]. Over the last 20 years, research has found that patients who report more trust in their physician and other health care providers are more engaged with their care [4], more likely to follow through on recommended care and medications [5–7], and often have better control of chronic conditions [8–10]. Trust in one's health provider is also related to better health care utilization, including greater continuity with a provider, not delaying care, and keeping appointments [11–13].

Fundamentally, trust in health providers is important to patients because patients turn to providers when they have a health problem that they are unable to independently address [14–16]. When seeking health care, patients are vulnerable, and need to rely on health providers' ability and commitment to address their health issues. Consistent with this, early measures

of trust, developed in the 1990s and 2000s, emphasize the concept of health care provider "fidelity" or working in the best interest of the patient [1,16–22]. Most of these measures also include dimensions of technical competence, confidentiality, and honesty. While early qualitative studies found that patient-doctor interpersonal dynamics were crucial for building trust [2,23], they were not the focus of most of these trust measures.

Two early trust measures, the Wake Forest Physician Trust Scale and the Trust in Physician Scale [1,19,22], are still commonly used [24–26]. More recently developed trust measures include a greater focus on patient-provider interpersonal dynamics, though they differ in how they do so. Hillen and colleagues, for example, developed a measure of trust in one's oncologist that added the domain of physician caring to those of fidelity, competence, and honesty [13]. The CAHPS Cultural Competency trust domain also emphasizes caring [27]. Bova and colleagues developed a measure that departs more substantially from earlier measures, with domains of interpersonal connection, respectful communication, and professional partnering [28].

There have been several recent experimental studies conducted in Europe using video vignettes to test whether specific physician behaviors impact peoples' trust in physicians. Hillen and colleagues found that videos of patient-oncologist interactions

* Corresponding author.
  E-mail addresses: Jessica.greene@baruch.cuny.edu (J. Greene),
cramos@urban.org (C. Ramos).

https://doi.org/10.1016/j.pec.2020.09.003
0738-3991/© 2020 Published by Elsevier B.V.

J. Greene, C. Ramos / Patient Education and Counseling 104 (2021) 1222–1228

emphasizing physician competence, honesty, and caring each resulted in higher trust assessments among viewers than a control vignette that emphasized none of these areas [29]. However, a follow up study by the same team found no differences in trust for those who viewed a video emphasizing all three dimensions compared to those who viewed a control video [30]. Another team conducted an experimental study that found higher trust among participants who watched a video of a doctor delivering a cancer diagnosis using caring and empathetic language compared to those who watched a video in which the doctors said the same message without caring language [31].

Recently, a working group of health care leaders and patient advocates in the United States have called for making health care-related trust measures a standard part of patient experience evaluation [32]. However, given the variation in how trust has previously been conceptualized and measured [33–35], it is important to better understand what patients believe builds their trust in health care providers. This mixed methods study uses qualitative methods to identify the health provider behaviors that patients report build trust, and quantitative methods to test the robustness of the findings using a national survey in the United States.

2. Methods

This mixed method study has two interrelated components [36]. The first was conducting semi-structured qualitative interviews to identify the key health care provider behaviors that patients reported build their trust, as well as those that lose their trust. Since the qualitative component was conducted with a relatively small, unrepresentative sample, the purpose of the study's second component was to validate the qualitative findings using a large nationally representative survey. We conducted secondary analysis of the Health Reform Monitoring Survey (HRMS) [37] to examine the relationship between trust and the

key components of trust identified in the qualitative component. We conducted the quantitative analysis for the full sample, and additionally conducted stratified analyses by race/ethnicity and household income to examine whether the findings were consistent across demographic subgroups.

2.1. Qualitative Methods

2.1.1. Interview Participants

We conducted 40 semi-structured telephone interviews [38] that each lasted approximately 20 minutes in May-July of 2018. Participants were respondents to the March 2018 HRMS, who had a usual health care provider and indicated on the survey a willingness to participate in a follow up telephone interview. We oversampled Black respondents and those with lower incomes (< = 138% federal poverty level) because of evidence that those groups have lower trust in health providers [39–42]. We additionally oversampled those reporting low trust in their usual provider in the HRMS.

The authors conducted 25 of the 40 interviews, and the rest were conducted by the first author's graduate students, who were studying qualitative research methods, and the second author's summer intern. The survey firm Ipsos reached out to participants to schedule the interviews, and provided the authors with interviewees' first name and telephone contact information. To maintain participants' confidentiality, identifying information was not retained nor connected to the transcripts or audio files. Participants gave verbal consent to participate, and earned $5 for participating. The study was approved by the human subjects committees of the Urban Institute and Baruch College.

2.1.2. Semi-Structured Interview Guide

The interview guide was developed to explore trust in participants' usual health care provider in several ways (we use the term "health care provider", though in interviews we used the

Table 1
Characteristics of the Study Participants.

	Interview Participants (n = 40)	Survey Participants (n = 6,392)
Gender		
Female	60.0	52.7
Male	40.0	47.3
Age		
18-34	12.5	29.9
35-49	42.5	30.1
50-64	45.0	40.0
Education		
<High School	7.5	8.5
High School Degree	30.0	26.1
Some College	35.0	29.7
College Graduate	27.5	35.7
Income (% of federal poverty level)		
≤138% FPL	47.5	19.2
>138%-<250% FPL	27.5	21.7
≥250% and <400% FPL	7.5	13.1
≥400% FPL	17.5	46.0
Race/ethnicity		
Black	30.0	11.5
Latinx	10.0	15.4
White	50.0	64.7
Other	7.5	8.4
Health Insurance		
Employer Sponsored	30.0	69.5
Medicaid	27.5	10.2
Medicare	20.0	4.8
Individual Market	10.0	8.5
Other/Unsure	10.0	2.7
Uninsured	10.0	4.2

Note: Several respondents had more than one type of insurance. Survey data was weighted.

J. Greene, C. Ramos / Patient Education and Counseling 104 (2021) 1222–1228

term "doctor" or "health care provider" depending on their type of usual clinician). First, participants were asked how much they trusted their usual provider, and then were asked an open-ended question about why they felt that way. For those with lower trust, we asked whether they had ever had a health provider who they strongly trusted and if so, what it was about the dynamic that made them trust the provider; and the reverse for those who did trust their health provider. Additionally, we asked for suggestions they would give a health provider for gaining patient trust and what to avoid that might lose patient trust. Interviewers used follow-up probes extensively to encourage participants to elaborate on their comments.

2.1.3. Interview Analysis

We used descriptive thematic analysis to analyze the interviews [43], all of which were audio recorded and transcribed verbatim. The two authors coded a handful of transcripts to identify the initial codes for the key provider behaviors that developed participants' trust. Each interview was then coded by the first author and one other researcher (either CR or one of two research assistants) to identify text blocks that corresponded to each code and to identify additional codes. The two authors reviewed the text related to each code to reconcile differences in coding and to determine sub-themes, which are detailed in the results section.

2.2. Quantitative Methods

2.2.1. Survey Participants

To test the robustness of the qualitative findings, we conducted secondary analysis of data from the March 2019 HRMS. The HRMS uses Ipsos' internet panel that is representative of English and Spanish speakers aged 18-64 in the United States, which has an approximately 62% rate of panel participation [37]. Of the 9,811 survey respondents, 6,666 (69%) had a usual health care provider. Our sample of 6,392 excluded those with missing data on key variables.

2.2.2. Quantitative Measures and Analysis

Trust was measured by asking respondents how much they agreed or disagreed with the following statement: "I trust my doctor (provider)" using a 5 point agree-disagree scale. We examined the relationship between health care provider trust

and the key provider behaviors identified in the qualitative component: communication, caring, and competence. All but one of the eight questions on communication, caring, and competence came from the CAHPS Cultural Competency survey (items are listed in Table 2) [19,27]. The items were all answered on Likert scales, so we used Spearman's rank order correlation to assess relationships. Since our qualitative data was from a sample that was disproportionally Black and low income, we also stratified our correlation analyses by race/ethnicity and family income to see whether our qualitative findings were consistent across subgroups.

3. Results

3.1. Interview Participant Characteristics

Qualitative interview participants were disproportionately **Black**, lower income, and female (Table 1). Almost half (48%) had incomes at or below 138% of the federal poverty level (FPL), and only a quarter had incomes at or above 250% FPL.

3.2. Importance of Trust and Its Key Dimensions

Participants almost all reported that trusting their usual health care provider was very important to them. A commonly expressed sentiment was, "I wouldn't go to a doctor I didn't trust." Those trusting their provider reported being more likely to share more personal information, listen to and follow through with the health provider's advice, and visit the provider regularly.

Overwhelmingly, patients described provider communication, caring, and competence as what builds their trust in health providers. These three dimensions of trust, which had considerable overlap, were each mentioned by 35 or more of the 40 respondents. In comparison, the areas of confidentiality, personal connection, and partnering, which have been the focus of several measures of trust [1,17,18,22,28], were each mentioned by fewer than one-quarter of participants. Health provider honesty and fidelity were described not as their own dimensions but as part of communication and caring respectively, as is described below.

3.2.1. Communication

Communication was described as crucial for building trust by all but two participants. The most common component detailed by

Table 2
Spearman's Rank Correlations between Trust in One's Usual Doctor (or Provider) and Items Related to Communication, Caring, and Competence, For Full Sample and Stratified by Race/Ethnicity and Family Income.

	Full Sample (n = 6,392)	Race/Ethnicity			Family Income			
		Black (n = 544)	Latinx (n = 812)	White (n = 4,609)	≤138% FPL (n = 943)	>138%-<250% FPL (n = 1,277)	≥250% and <400% FPL (n = 956)	≥400% FPL (3,087)
Communication								
My doctor/provider listens carefully to what I have to say	0.69	0.65	0.71	0.70	0.73	0.72	0.66	0.68
My doctor/provider explains things in a way that is easy for me to understand	0.65	0.65	0.66	0.65	0.68	0.68	0.63	0.63
My doctor/provider tells the truth, even if it is bad news	0.62	0.64	0.61	0.62	0.66	0.65	0.61	0.60
Caring								
My doctor/provider cares about me as a person	0.68	0.69	0.66	0.68	0.70	0.72	0.69	0.65
My doctor/provider takes my questions and concerns seriously	0.71	0.69	0.66	0.73	0.74	0.73	0.70	0.70
[Reverse] My doctor/provider does not spend enough time with me	0.52	0.52	0.53	0.51	0.53	0.55	0.55	0.49
Competence								
I have confidence in the medical care provided by my doctor/provider	0.76	0.74	0.75	0.77	0.74	0.78	0.76	0.75
My doctor/provider is thorough and careful	0.73	0.70	0.72	0.74	0.76	0.75	0.70	0.72

Notes: All correlations have p-values <.01. For those whose usual clinician was not a doctor, the term "provider" was used rather than "doctor." FPL is federal poverty level.

J. Greene, C. Ramos / Patient Education and Counseling 104 (2021) 1222–1228

participants was health providers' listening. A 38-year-old man described having trust in his new provider: "We communicated and I would tell him everything about me from head to toe. He really listened." Several people who described having low trust in their provider said it was because, "I just . . . don't feel listened to," or "He just dismisses my questions."

Participants also stressed the importance of health providers providing detailed explanations. Receiving comprehensive information was highly valued because it enabled participants to understand their condition and the approach to their care. A 38-year-old woman described the importance of her provider preparing her for cancer treatment: "She made me feel comfortable every step of the way. She explained everything to me thoroughly and . . . told me what to expect. So there were no surprises as I was dealing with my treatment." A 54-year-old man described the reverse resulting in lower trust. At a recent visit, his cardiologist said his heart looked good, but wanted to him to wear a heart monitor for a few weeks. "I was like, 'Well, why do I need to wear this heart monitor if everything's fine?' He didn't answer."

A key component of providing detailed explanations was providers being able to speak in a way that was clear "for people that don't have a medical degree." Participants also repeatedly emphasized the importance of providers being up front and honest. A 38-year old woman said, "Don't hide anything, don't down play it, just tell me however good or however bad it is. Just be open with me," and a 63-year old woman commented, "I like absolute truth and details."

3.2.2. Caring

All but five participants reported that a key way health providers earned their trust was through showing caring; specifically by showing interest in patients as individuals, valuing patients' experience, and being committed to solving patients' health issues. Being treated as an individual was very important to participants. A 36-year-old woman described a health provider that she highly trusted: "I could tell she really cared about me personally for who I was. I was not just a faceless patient."

Valuing patient experience was another way that providers show their patients that they care. A 55-year-old man described his doctor as "believing in me" when she, unlike his prior provider, changed his medication in response to his concerns about its effectiveness. Similarly a 35-year-old woman described how important it was that her health provider "did not question my perception" after having an uncomfortable interaction with a specialist.

Participants with strong trust in their health providers often described their provider as being committed to solving their health concerns. A 53-year-old woman explained, "I know that she's going to do her best to help me get through whatever is going on . . . She's going to just try to help me." For some respondents, this dedication to helping patients with their health conditions was described as one end of the caring spectrum in contrast to provider self-interest, at the other end. A 64-year-old man explained, "You have some doctors that are really there to help you and then you have some doctors that they just care about their timeshare and the bottom line."

One way that participants detected that their provider cared about them and their health was the amount of time spent together during a visit. A 57-year-old woman explained, "The doctor spends a good amount of time with me, at least 20 minutes or so in each visit. He seems to be concerned about my health. He is genuinely interested."

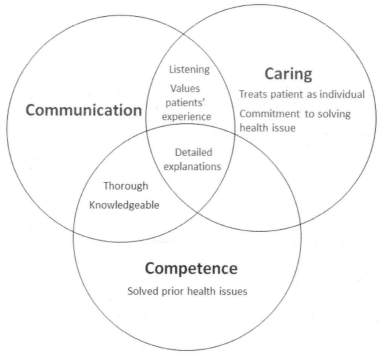

Fig. 1. Qualitative Themes and Subthemes, and How They Are Overlapping.

J. Greene, C. Ramos / Patient Education and Counseling 104 (2021) 1222–1228

3.2.3. Competence

All but one participant described health provider competence as being important for developing trust. Competence was described as a provider being knowledgeable, thorough, and solving their prior health issues.

Health care providers were perceived as knowledgeable based upon their ability to provide information and context about patients' health issues. A 28-year-old woman described the physician she strongly trusted: "He is very competent. Able to express himself very well, and is knowledgeable about the treatment process and can help provide clarity on the illness that I'm having." Others described providers they trusted in the following ways: "she knows what she's talking about" and "he is very astute."

Being thorough was frequently mentioned as a key element of competence, and thoroughness was referred to in examining, testing, and asking questions. A 38-year-old man with diabetes described his physician's thoroughness as a key factor in why he trusted him: "When I go see him . . . he goes through everything. My medications are sitting on the counter and he goes one by one and we discuss everything."

Another way that participants detected competence was when the health provider had solved a prior health issue. A 54-year-old man described trusting his provider because, "...I've had some health issues, he's always got them under control," whereas a 50-year-old woman with low trust in her physician described, "I feel like I'm just being a guinea pig as we eliminate things."

3.2.4. Overlapping Domains

The three dimensions of trust were overlapping, and not mutually exclusive (Fig. 1). For example, providing detailed explanations, which is a key component of communication, also demonstrates that a provider is caring and is competent. Listening, also a key component of communication, also shows caring. Competence and caring are also overlapping, in particular when a provider is thorough it suggests both clinical competence to patients as well as caring, through interest in the patient.

3.3. Survey Participant Characteristics

Table 1 shows the characteristics of those in the national sample who had a usual health care provider. For the vast majority (89%), their usual provider was a physician and the remaining 11% had another type of usual health provider. The sample was close to evenly split by gender (53% female). A third (36%) had a college education and almost half (46%) had incomes ≥400% FPL.

3.4. Quantitative Results

Almost all respondents (90%) trusted their usual health provider, with 62% reporting strong trust and 29% some trust (not shown). Only 2% reported not trusting their provider and 8% reported neither trusting nor distrusting their provider.

Trust in one's health provider was highly correlated with the communication, caring, and competence items (Table 2). The strongest correlations were with competence; specifically having "confidence in the medical care provided by my doctor/provider" (0.76) and "my doctor/provider is thorough and careful" (0.73). Trust was also highly correlated with caring, particularly "my doctor/provider takes my questions and concerns seriously" (0.71). The communication item, "My doctor/provider listens carefully to what I have to say" was also highly correlated with trust (0.69). The lowest correlation was with "my doctor/provider does not spend enough time with me" (0.52), which was reverse coded.

Stratified analyses show that trust was highly correlated with these eight items for all the racial/ethnic and income subgroups. The two competence items had the highest correlation with trust for each of the subgroups, and the item with the lowest correlation was consistent across each group. Across subgroups, the correlation coefficients for each of the items were very similar, differing between .04 and .08.

4. Discussion and Conclusion

4.1. Discussion

Nine out of 10 people in the United States who had a regular physician or other health care provider, reported having strong trust in their provider. What builds their trust is a combination of the health provider communicating effectively, caring about them and their health, and demonstrating competence. For communication, participants stressed the importance of being listened to and having detailed and honest explanations about their health issues. Caring was described as providers treating them as an individual, valuing their experience, and showing commitment to solving their health issues. Competence was detected when health providers were knowledgeable, thorough, and able to solve health issues. These three dimensions of trust, which were identified through qualitative interviews, were found to be highly correlated with trust in a recent national survey, and were consistently related to trust regardless of participants' race/ethnicity or income.

Our findings are consistent with a number of qualitative research studies [2,23,44,45] and quantitative studies [29,31,46], including one review of literature on cancer patients' trust in their physician that found trust was enhanced by perceived physician competence and patient-centered communication [35]. However, our findings are less consistent with how the most utilized trust measures are conceptualized [1,19,22]. The key dimension in most trust measures is fidelity, or working in the best interest of the patient. Rather than fidelity, what participants described as key to building trust was feeling that their health provider cared about them. Caring was seen as the high end of the continuum, which at the low end was provider self-interest. When a health care provider demonstrates caring for a patient, the provider is assumed to be acting in the patient's best interest; however, the reverse is not necessarily true. When authors have considered health provider caring as an element of trust, it has often been a component of fidelity [1,15], while others have conceptualized the two concepts separately [13].

Other disconnects between our findings and existing trust measures include that effective communication is included in few provider trust measures [21,28]. And while existing measures typically do include a dimension of honesty [1,13,18–22], we found honesty to be one element of the broader theme of communication. We found only one health care provider trust scale that included the three dimensions identified in our qualitative research, but it is long (51 items) and includes topics that were not widely endorsed, like confidentiality. [21]

Our findings should be interpreted in light of the study's limitations. The qualitative interviews were conducted with a disproportionately vulnerable sample. That was purposeful since people from racial and ethnic minority backgrounds and with lower incomes have often reported lower trust in their physicians than whites [39–42], and we wanted to better understand trust from their perspective. Our quantitative component suggests that our findings are consistent across racial/ethnic and income groups. Another limitation is that we were not able to quantitatively test every element of our qualitative findings. While we had relevant items related to communication, caring, and competence; we did not have items specific to some subdimensions like a provider's commitment to addressing the patient's health issues. Additionally, one item, related to the provider spending enough time with the patient, was phrased in the negative, which may have reduced its

J. Greene, C. Ramos / Patient Education and Counseling 104 (2021) 1222–1228

correlation to trust. Finally, this study examined only interpersonal trust with health care providers, and excluded the broader literature on trust that includes trust in health care institutions, and other areas like medical technology and medical research [33,47–49].

4.2. Practice Implications

Since trust is related to better patient health-related behaviors and utilization, it is important for health care providers to actively listen, provide detailed explanations, show care and concern for patients and their health, and demonstrate their knowledge. Making time in clinical practice for effective communication and caring, however, can be challenging for health providers. In a recent JAMA article, a neurology resident described how her medical training had resulted in her becoming a worse listener and less caring [50]. Future research should test whether strategies to improve health provider communication, like motivational interviewing [51], impact patient trust and health outcomes. Further, building trusting relationships with patients may not only have positive impacts on patients. Trusting patient-provider relationships may improve health care provider wellbeing, job fulfillment, as well as care team dynamics [3,50], and these relationships also warrant future investigation.

4.3. Conclusion

Respondents in this study reported that trusting their health care provider was crucial for them to visit the provider, share personal information with the provider and follow through with the provider's advice. To earn their trust, participants said that health providers need to communicate effectively, express that they care about their patients and their patients' health, and demonstrate competence. This study provides a framework for future measures of trust, both in areas that have been well studied, like trust in health providers, as well as in areas where there has been less research, like trust in pediatricians [34], and trust in health care institutions [33].

5. Support

This research was funded by the Robert Wood Johnson Foundation.

CRediT authorship contribution statement

Jessica Greene: Conceptualization, Methodology, Investigation, Writing - original draft. **Christal Ramos:** Conceptualization, Investigation, Project administration, Writing - review & editing.

Declaration of Competing Interest

The authors report no declarations of interest.

Acknowledgements

We would like to thank the Urban Institutes' Nina Bart, Graeme Peterson, Dulce Gonzalez, Sophia Yin, and Malvika Govil for their contributions to data analysis. We would also like to thank the students from Baruch College's Marxe School of Public and International Affairs for conducting a number of the semi-structured interviews.

References

[1] L.A. Anderson, R.F. Dedrick, Development of the Trust in Physician Scale: A Measure to Assess Interpersonal Trust in Patient-Physician Relationships, Psychol. Rep. 67 (1990) 1091–1100, doi:http://dx.doi.org/10.2466/pr0.1990.67.3f.1091.

[2] D.H. Thom, B. Campbell, Patient-physician trust: an exploratory study, J. Fam. Pract 44 (1997) 169–177. (accessed October 6, 2017) http://go.galegroup.com/ps/anonymous?id=GALE%7CA19181949&sid=googleScholar&v=2.1&it=r&linkaccess=fulltext&issn=00943509&p=AONE&sw=w&authCount=1&isAnonymousEntry=true.

[3] C.A. Pellegrini, Trust: The Keystone of the Patient-Physician Relationship, J. Am. Coll. Surg. 224 (2017) 95–102, doi:http://dx.doi.org/10.1016/j.jamcollsurg.2016.10.032.

[4] E.R. Becker, D.W. Roblin, Translating Primary Care Practice Climate into Patient Activation: The Role of Patient Trust in Physician 46 (2008) 795–805, doi:http://dx.doi.org/10.1097/MLR.0b013e31817919c0. http://journals.lww.com/lww-medicalcare/Fulltext/2008/08000/Translating_Primary_Care_Practice_Climate_into.6.aspx.

[5] A. Braksmajer, T.M. Fedor, S.-R. Chen, R. Corales, S. Holt, W. Valenti, J.M. McMahon, Willingness to Take PrEP for HIV Prevention: The Combined Effects of Race/Ethnicity and Provider Trust, AIDS Educ. Prev. 30 (2018) 1–12, doi:http://dx.doi.org/10.1521/aeap.2018.30.1.1.

[6] S. Gupta, A.T. Brenner, N. Ratanawongsa, J.M. Inadomi, Patient Trust in Physician Influences Colorectal Cancer Screening in Low-Income Patients, Am. J. Prev. Med 47 (2014) 417–423, doi:http://dx.doi.org/10.1016/J.AMEPRE.2014.04.020.

[7] N. Ratanawongsa, A.J. Karter, M.M. Parker, C.R. Lyles, M. Heisler, H.H. Moffet, N. Adler, E.M. Warton, D. Schillinger, Communication and Medication Refill Adherence, JAMA Intern. Med. 173 (2013) 210, doi:http://dx.doi.org/10.1001/jamainternmed.2013.1216.

[8] J. Birkhäuer, J. Gaab, J. Kossowsky, S. Hasler, P. Krummenacher, C. Werner, H. Gerger, Trust in the health care professional and health outcome: A meta-analysis, PLoS One. 12 (2017)e0170988, doi:http://dx.doi.org/10.1371/journal.pone.0170988.

[9] A. Fernandez, H. Seligman, J. Quan, R.J. Stern, E.A. Jacobs, Associations between aspects of culturally competent care and clinical outcomes among patients with diabetes, Med. Care. 50 (2012) S74–79, doi:http://dx.doi.org/10.1097/MLR.0b013e3182641110.

[10] A. Schoenthaler, E. Montague, L. Baier Manwell, R. Brown, M.D. Schwartz, M. Linzer, Patient–physician racial/ethnic concordance and blood pressure control: the role of trust and medication adherence, Ethn. Health. 19 (2014) 565–578, doi:http://dx.doi.org/10.1080/13557858.2013.857764.

[11] S. Mollborn, I. Stepanikova, K.S. Cook, Delayed Care and Unmet Needs among Health Care System Users: When Does Fiduciary Trust in a Physician Matter? Health Serv. Res. 40 (2005) 1898–1917, doi:http://dx.doi.org/10.1111/j.1475-6773.2005.00457.x.

[12] G.C. Nguyen, T.A. LaVeist, M.L. Harris, L.W. Datta, T.M. Bayless, S.R. Brant, Patient trust-in-physician and race are predictors of adherence to medical management in inflammatory bowel disease, Inflamm. Bowel Dis 15 (2009) 1233–1239, doi:http://dx.doi.org/10.1002/ibd.20883.

[13] M.A. Hillen, P.N. Butow, M.H.N. Tattersall, G. Hruby, F.M. Boyle, J. Vardy, B.L. Kallimanis-King, H.C.J.M. de Haes, E.M.A. Smets, Validation of the English version of the Trust in Oncologist Scale (TiOS), Patient Educ. Couns 91 (2013) 25–28, doi:http://dx.doi.org/10.1016/J.PEC.2012.11.004.

[14] D.H. Thom, M.A. Hall, L.G. Pawlson, Measuring patients' trust in physicians when assessing quality of care, Health Aff. (Millwood). 23 (2004) 124–132, doi:http://dx.doi.org/10.1377/HLTHAFF.23.4.124.

[15] M.A. Hall, E. Dugan, B. Zheng, A.K. Mishra, Trust in Physicians and Medical Institutions: What Is It, Can It Be Measured, and Does It Matter? Milbank Q. 79 (2001) 613–639, doi:http://dx.doi.org/10.1111/1468-0009.00223.

[16] L.E. Egede, C. Ellis, Development and Testing of the Multidimensional Trust in Health Care Systems Scale, J. Gen. Intern. Med. 23 (2008) 808–815, doi:http://dx.doi.org/10.1007/s11606-008-0613-1.

[17] A.C. Kao, D.C. Green, N.A. Davis, J.P. Koplan, P.D. Cleary, Patients' trust in their physicians: effects of choice, continuity, and payment method, J. Gen. Intern. Med. 13 (1998) 681–686, doi:http://dx.doi.org/10.1046/J.1525-1497.1998.00204.X.

[18] D.G. Safran, M. Kosinski, A.R. Tarlov, W.H. Rogers, D.H. Taira, N. Lieberman, J.E. Ware, The Primary Care Assessment Survey: tests of data quality and measurement performance, Med. Care. 36 (1998) 728–739. (accessed March 11, 2019) http://www.ncbi.nlm.nih.gov/pubmed/9596063.

[19] M.A. Hall, B. Zheng, E. Dugan, F. Camacho, K.E. Kidd, A. Mishra, R. Balkrishnan, Measuring Patients' Trust in their Primary Care Providers, Med. Care Res. Rev. 59 (2002) 293–318, doi:http://dx.doi.org/10.1177/1077558702059003004.

[20] E. Dugan, F. Trachtenberg, M.A. Hall, Development of abbreviated measures to assess patient trust in a physician, a health insurer, and the medical profession, BMC Health Serv. Res 5 (64) (2005), doi:http://dx.doi.org/10.1186/1472-6963-5-64.

[21] B. Leisen, M.R. Hyman, An Improved Scale for Assessing Patients' Trust in Their Physician, Health Mark. Q. 19 (2001) 23–42, doi:http://dx.doi.org/10.1300/J026v19n01_03.

[22] D.H. Thom, K.M. Ribisl, A.L. Stewart, D.A. Luke, Further validation and reliability testing of the Trust in Physician Scale. The Stanford Trust Study Physicians, Med. Care 37 (1999) 510–517. (accessed March 11, 2019) http://www.ncbi.nlm.nih.gov/pubmed/10335753.

[23] D. Mechanic, S. Meyer, Concepts of trust among patients with serious illness, Soc. Sci. Med. 51 (2000) 657–668, doi:http://dx.doi.org/10.1016/S0277-9536(00)00014-9.

1228 *J. Greene, C. Ramos / Patient Education and Counseling 104 (2021) 1222–1228*

[24] J. Tsai, L. Gelberg, R.A. Rosenheck, Changes in Physical Health After Supported Housing: Results from the Collaborative Initiative to End Chronic Homelessness, J. Gen. Intern. Med. 34 (2019) 1703–1708, doi:http://dx.doi.org/10.1007/s11606-019-05070-y.

[25] R.J. Kovacs, M. Lagarde, J. Cairns, Measuring patient trust: Comparing measures from a survey and an economic experiment, Health Econ 28 (2019) 641–652, doi:http://dx.doi.org/10.1002/hec.3870.

[26] G.P. Kanter, D. Carpenter, L.S. Lehmann, M.M. Mello, US Nationwide Disclosure of Industry Payments and Public Trust in Physicians, JAMA Netw. Open. 2 (2019)e191947, doi:http://dx.doi.org/10.1001/jamanetworkopen.2019.1947.

[27] R. Weech-Maldonado, A. Carle, B. Weidmer, M. Hurtado, Q. Ngo-Metzger, R.D. Hays, The Consumer Assessment of Healthcare Providers and Systems (CAHPS) cultural competence (CC) item set, Med. Care. 50 (2012) S22–31, doi:http://dx.doi.org/10.1097/MLR.0b013e318263134b.

[28] C. Bova, P.S. Route, K. Fennie, W. Ettinger, G.W. Manchester, B. Weinstein, Measuring patient-provider trust in a primary care population: Refinement of the health care relationship trust scale, Res. Nurs. Health. 35 (2012) 397–408, doi:http://dx.doi.org/10.1002/nur.21484.

[29] M.A. Hillen, H.C.J.M. de Haes, L.J.A. Stalpers, J.H.G. Klinkenbijl, E.H. Eddes, P.N. Butow, J. van der Vloodt, H.W.M. van Laarhoven, E.M.A. Smets, How can communication by oncologists enhance patients' trust? An experimental study, Ann. Oncol. 25 (2014) 896–901, doi:http://dx.doi.org/10.1093/annonc/mdu027.

[30] N.M. Medendorp, L.N.C. Visser, M.A. Hillen, J.C.J.M. de Haes, E.M.A. Smets, How oncologists' communication improves (analogue) patients' recall of information. A randomized video-vignettes study, Patient Educ. Couns 100 (2017) 1338–1344, doi:http://dx.doi.org/10.1016/J.PEC.2017.02.012.

[31] J. Zwingmann, W.F. Baile, J.W. Schmier, J. Bernhard, M. Keller, Effects of patient-centered communication on anxiety, negative affect, and trust in the physician in delivering a cancer diagnosis: A randomized, experimental study, Cancer. 123 (2017) 3167–3175, doi:http://dx.doi.org/10.1002/cncr.30694.

[32] T.H. Lee, E.A. McGlynn, D.G. Safran, A Framework for Increasing Trust Between Patients and the Organizations That Care for Them, JAMA. 321 (2019) 539, doi:http://dx.doi.org/10.1001/jama.2018.19186.

[33] S. Ozawa, P. Sripad, How do you measure trust in the health system? A systematic review of the literature, Soc. Sci. Med. 91 (2013) 10–14, doi:http://dx.doi.org/10.1016/J.SOCSCIMED.2013.05.005.

[34] B. Sisk, J.N. Baker, A model of interpersonal trust, credibility, and relationship maintenance, Pediatrics. 144 (2019), doi:http://dx.doi.org/10.1542/peds.2019-1319.

[35] M.A. Hillen, H.C.J.M. De Haes, E.M.A. Smets, Cancer patients' trust in their physician - A review, Psychooncology. 20 (2011) 227–241, doi:http://dx.doi.org/10.1002/pon.1745.

[36] M.D. Fetters, L.A. Curry, J.W. Creswell, Achieving integration in mixed methods designs - Principles and practices, Health Serv. Res. 48 (2013) 2134–2156, doi:http://dx.doi.org/10.1111/1475-6773.12117.

[37] S.K. Long, G.M. Kenney, S. Zuckerman, D.E. Goin, D. Wissoker, F. Blavin, L.J. Blumberg, L. Clemans-Cope, J. Holahan, K. Hempstead, The Health Reform Monitoring Survey: Addressing Data Gaps To Provide Timely Insights Into The Affordable Care Act, Health Aff. 33 (2014) 161–167, doi:http://dx.doi.org/10.1377/hlthaff.2013.0934.

[38] M. Cachia, L. Millward, The telephone medium and semi-structured interviews: A complementary fit, Qual. Res. Organ. Manag. An Int. J. 6 (2011) 265–277, doi:http://dx.doi.org/10.1108/17465641111188420.

[39] K.D. Martin, D.L. Roter, M.C. Beach, K.A. Carson, L.A. Cooper, Physician communication behaviors and trust among black and white patients with hypertension, Med. Care. 51 (2013) 151–157, doi:http://dx.doi.org/10.1097/MLR.0b013e31827632a2.

[40] I.V. Blair, J.F. Steiner, D.L. Fairclough, R. Hanratty, D.W. Price, H.K. Hirsh, L.A. Wright, M. Bronsert, E. Karimkhani, D.J. Magid, E.P. Havranek, Clinicians' implicit ethnic/racial bias and perceptions of care among Black and Latino patients, Ann. Fam. Med. 11 (2013) 43–52, doi:http://dx.doi.org/10.1370/afm.1442.

[41] S. Hwang, R DV, S. Kerr, T. Heeren, E. Colson, M. Corwin, Predictors of Maternal Trust in Doctors About Advice on Infant Care Practices: The SAFE Study, Acad. Pediatr. 17 (2017) 762–769, doi:http://dx.doi.org/10.1016/J.ACAP.2017.03.005.

[42] V.S. Freimuth, A.M. Jamison, J. An, G.R. Hancock, S.C. Quinn, Determinants of trust in the flu vaccine for African Americans and Whites, Soc. Sci. Med. 193 (2017) 70–79, doi:http://dx.doi.org/10.1016/J.SOCSCIMED.2017.10.001.

[43] M. Sandelowski, What's in a name? Qualitative description revisited, Res. Nurs. Heal. 33 (2010) 77–84, doi:http://dx.doi.org/10.1002/nur.20362.

[44] M.A. Hillen, A.T. Onderwater, M.C.B. van Zwieten, H.C.J.M. de Haes, E.M.A. Smets, Disentangling cancer patients' trust in their oncologist: a qualitative study, Psychooncology. 21 (2012) 392–399, doi:http://dx.doi.org/10.1002/pon.1910.

[45] B.N. Dang, R.A. Westbrook, S.M. Njue, T.P. Giordano, Building trust and rapport early in the new doctor-patient relationship: a longitudinal qualitative study, BMC Med. Educ 17 (2017) 1–10, doi:http://dx.doi.org/10.1186/s12909-017-0868-5.

[46] D.H. Thom, Physician Behaviors that Predict Patient Trust, J. Fam. Pract 50 (2001) 323–323. http://go.galegroup.com/ps/anonymous?id=GALE%7CA74292253&sid=googleScholar&v=2.1&it=r&linkaccess=fulltext&issn=00943509&p=AONE&sw=w&authCount=1&isAnonymousEntry=true (accessed October 7, 2017).

[47] Z. Zhang, T.W. Bickmore, M.K. Paasche-Orlow, Perceived organizational affiliation and its effects on patient trust: Role modeling with embodied conversational agents, Patient Educ. Couns 100 (2017) 1730–1737, doi:http://dx.doi.org/10.1016/j.pec.2017.03.017.

[48] E. Montague, Validation of a trust in medical technology instrument, Appl. Ergon. 41 (2010) 812–821, doi:http://dx.doi.org/10.1016/j.apergo.2010.01.009.

[49] P. Crits-Christoph, A. Rieger, A. Gaines, M.B.C. Gibbons, Trust and respect in the patient-clinician relationship: Preliminary development of a new scale, BMC Psychol. 7 (2019) 91, doi:http://dx.doi.org/10.1186/s40359-019-0347-3.

[50] A. Goss, How Becoming a Doctor Made Me a Worse Listener, JAMA. 323 (2020) 1041–1042.

[51] L.L. Söderlund, M.B. Madson, S. Rubak, P. Nilsen, A systematic review of motivational interviewing training for general health care practitioners, Patient Educ. Couns 84 (2011) 16–26, doi:http://dx.doi.org/10.1016/j.pec.2010.06.025.

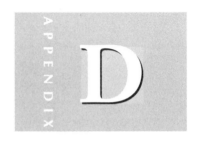

Appraisal Guidelines

KEY PRINCIPLES FOR CRITICAL APPRAISAL

Key Principles for Critically Appraising Quantitative and Qualitative Studies

- *Read and critically appraise the entire study.* A research critical appraisal involves examining the quality of all aspects of the research report.
- *Examine the organization and presentation of the research report.* A well-prepared report is concise, complete, logically organized, and clearly presented. It does not include excessive jargon that is difficult to read. The references need to be current, complete, and presented in a consistent format.
- *Examine the significance of the problem studied for nursing practice.* Nursing studies need to be focused on significant problems if a sound knowledge base is to be developed for evidence-based nursing practice.
- *Indicate the type of study conducted and identify the steps or elements of the study.* This might be done as an initial critical appraisal of a study, indicating your knowledge of the different types of quantitative and qualitative studies and the elements included in these studies.
- *Identify the strengths and weaknesses of a study.* All studies have strengths and weaknesses. Review the limitations identified by the researchers in a study and how they were managed to ensure the credibility of the findings.
- *Be objective and realistic in identifying the study's strengths and weaknesses.* Be balanced in your critical appraisal of a study. Try not to be overly critical in identifying a study's weaknesses or overly flattering in identifying the strengths. Take the limitations identified by the researchers into consideration but do not repeat these in your critique.
- *Provide specific examples of the strengths and weaknesses of a study.* Examples provide evidence for your critical appraisal of a study's strengths and weaknesses.
- *Provide a rationale for your critical appraisal comments.* Include justifications for your critical appraisal and document your ideas with sources from the current literature.
- *Evaluate the quality of the study.* Describe the credibility of the findings, consistency of the findings with those from previous studies, and appropriateness of the study conclusions.
- *Discuss the usefulness of the findings for practice.* The findings from the study need to be linked to the findings of previous studies and examined for use in clinical practice.

CRITICAL APPRAISAL GUIDELINES

Step 1: Identifying the Steps of the Study

1. Introduction
   a. Was the article title clear? Does the title indicate the type of study conducted (descriptive, correlational, quasi-experimental, or experimental), variables, and population (Gray & Grove, 2021; Kazdin, 2017; Shadish et al., 2002)?
   b. Did the abstract include the purpose, type of design, sample, and intervention (if applicable) and present key results and conclusions (APA, 2020)?

2. State the problem.
   a. Did the researchers provide the significance of the problem, such as number of people affected, its importance to nursing practice, and cost incurred?
   b. Did the researchers provide the background of the problem?
   c. Was there a clear problem statement (see Chapter 5)?

3. State the purpose.

4. Examine the literature review.
   a. Does the literature review cite previous studies and theory for the framework?
   b. Are the references current? Number and percentage of sources in the last 10 years and in the last 5 years? (see Chapter 6; Jones et al., 2020)

5. Examine the study framework or theoretical perspective.
   a. Is the framework explicitly expressed, or must you extract the framework from statements in the introduction or literature review of the study?
   b. Were the concepts and at least one relationship identified, providing a theoretical basis for the study (Chinn et al., 2022; Smith & Liehr, 2018)?

6. List the research objectives, questions, and/or hypotheses guiding the study.

7. Identify which of the following types of variable were included in the study: independent, dependent, and/or research variables. A study with an independent variable also includes dependent variables. Research variables are commonly included in descriptive and some correlational studies (see Chapter 5).
   What were the conceptual and operational definitions of two study variables or concepts that were identified in the objectives, questions, or hypotheses? If these are not stated, you need to identify and define two variables in the study purpose.

8. Identify attribute or demographic variables.
   a. What person-related demographic variables were measured, such as income, age, and marital status?
   b. Were other demographic variables measured, such as diagnosis, time since diagnosis, and prescriptions identified?

9. Identify the research design.
   a. What is the specific design of the study (see Chapter 8; Gray & Grove, 2021; Kazdin, 2017; Shadish et al., 2002)?
   b. Does the study include a treatment or intervention? If so, identify the intervention.
   c. If the study has more than one group, how were participants assigned to groups?

10. Describe the sample and setting.
    a. What were the inclusion and exclusion criteria for the sample (see Chapter 9)?
    b. What specific type of probability or nonprobability sampling method was used to obtain the sample? Did the researchers identify the sampling frame for the study?
    c. What was the sample size? Discuss the refusal rate and percentage, and include the rationale for refusal if presented in the article. Identify if power analysis was used to determine sample size (Aberson, 2019).
    d. What was the attrition of the sample (number and percentage) for the study?
    e. What were the characteristics of the sample?
    f. What was the study setting?

11. Identify the ethical considerations.
    a. Was the study reviewed by an institutional or ethical board?
    b. What was the process for informed consent?

12. Identify at least two measurement strategies used in the study. Include the essential information listed below for a scale or physiological measure in a table format.

Variable Measured	Name of Measurement Method	Type of Method and Level of Measurement	Reliability or Precision	Validity or Accuracy

a. What were the two key variables that were measured?
b. What was the name of each measurement method, such as the Spiritual Well-Being Scale or adherence questionnaire?
c. What type of measurement strategy was used (e.g., Likert scale, visual analog scale, physiological measure, or existing database) (Bandalos, 2018; DeVellis, 2017; Waltz et al., 2017)?
d. What was the level of measurement (nominal, ordinal, interval, or ratio) achieved by the measurement method used in the study (Grove & Cipher, 2020)?
e. What information was provided about the reliability of each scale based on previous studies and for this study? What information was provided about the precision of each physiological measure (Bandalos, 2018; Bialocerkowski et al., 2010; Ryan-Wenger, 2017; Waltz et al., 2017)?
f. What information was provided about the validity of each scale (DeVellis, 2017) and the accuracy of physiological measures (Ryan-Wenger, 2017)?

Example Table of Measurement Methods

Variable Measured	Name of Measurement Method	Type of Method and Level of Measurement	Reliability or Precision	Validity or Accuracy
Depression	Beck Depression Inventory	Likert Scale Interval-level data	Cronbach's alphas of 0.82–0.92 from previous studies and 0.84 for this study. Reading level at sixth grade.	*Content validity* from concept analysis, literature review, and reviews of experts. *Construct validity:* convergent validity of 0.04 with Zung Depression Scale. *Predictive validity* of patients' future depression episodes. *Successive use validity* with previous studies and this study.

Variable Measured	Name of Measurement Method	Type of Method and Level of Measurement	Reliability or Precision	Validity or Accuracy
Blood pressure (BP)	Omron BP equipment	Physiological measure Ratio-level data	Test-retest values of BPs in previous studies. BP equipment new and recalibrated every 100 BP readings.	Documented accuracy of systolic and diastolic BPs to 1 mm Hg by company developing Omron BP cuff. Designated protocol for taking BP (Whelton et al., 2018). Average three BP readings to determine most accurate BP.

13. Identify the procedures for data collection.

14. Describe the statistical analyses used.
    a. What statistical procedures were conducted to describe the sample?
    b. Was the level of significance or alpha identified? If so, indicate what it was (0.05, 0.01, or 0.001).
    c. Identify the statistical procedures conducted to address the research objectives, questions, or hypotheses (see Chapter 11; Grove & Cipher, 2020; Kim et al., 2022; Leedy & Ormrod, 2019).
    d. Complete a table with the following information from the appraised study: (1) identify the focus (description, relationships, or differences) for each analysis technique, (2) list the statistical technique performed, (3) list the statistic, (4) provide the specific results, and (5) identify the probability (*p*) of the statistical significance achieved by the result (Grove & Cipher, 2020; Kim et al., 2022; Leedy & Ormrod, 2019).

Example Table of Statistical Analyses

Purpose of Analysis	Analysis Technique	Statistic	Results	Probability
Description of subjects' pulse rate	Mean Standard deviation Range	M SD $Range$	71.52 5.62 58–97	
Difference between adult males and females for oxygen saturation	t-test	t	3.75	$p = 0.001$
Differences of diet group, exercise group, and comparison group for pounds lost in adolescents	Analysis of variance	F	4.27	$p = 0.04$

Purpose of Analysis	Analysis Technique	Statistic	Results	Probability
Relationship of depression and anxiety in the elderly	Pearson correlation coefficient	*r*	0.46	$p = 0.03$

15. What were the findings of the study? Identify two findings discussed by the researchers.

16. What study limitations did the researcher identify?

17. Did the researcher generalize the findings?

18. What were the implications of the findings for nursing practice?

19. What suggestions for further study were identified?

20. What conclusions did the researchers identify?

Step 2: Determining Study Strengths and Weaknesses

1. Research problem and purpose
   a. Is the problem significant for nursing (Gallagher-Ford et al., 2020; O'Mathúna & Fineout-Overholt, 2019)?
   b. Does the purpose narrow and clarify the focus of the study?
   c. Was the study feasible to conduct in terms of money commitment; the researchers' expertise; and availability of participants, facilities, and equipment (see Chapter 5)?

2. Review of literature
   a. Is the literature review organized to demonstrate the progressive development of evidence from previous research?
   b. Does the summary of the literature review identify what is known and not known about the research problem and provide direction for the formation of the purpose (Grainger, 2021; Jones et al., 2020)?

3. Study framework
   a. Is the framework presented with clarity? If a model or conceptual map of the framework is present, is it adequate to explain the phenomenon of concern?
   b. If a proposition from a theory is to be tested, is the proposition clearly identified and linked to the study hypotheses (Chinn et al., 2022; Gray & Grove, 2021)?
   c. Is the framework related to the study findings?

4. Research objectives, questions, or hypotheses
   a. Are the objectives, questions, or hypotheses expressed clearly and logically linked to the purpose (Gray & Grove, 2021)?
   b. Are hypotheses stated to direct the conduct of quasi-experimental and experimental research (Kazdin, 2017; Shadish et al., 2002)?
   c. Are the objectives, questions, or hypotheses logically linked to the study results (Grove & Cipher, 2020; Kim et al., 2022)?

5. Variables
   a. Are the variables reflective of the concepts identified in the framework?
   b. Are the variables clearly defined (conceptually and operationally) and based on previous theories and research (Chinn et al., 2022; Smith & Liehr, 2018)?
   c. Is the conceptual definition of a variable consistent with the operational definition?

6. Design
   a. Is the design used in the study the most appropriate design to address the research purpose and to obtain essential data (Gray & Grove, 2021; Kazdin, 2017; Shadish et al., 2002)?
   b. Does the design provide a means to examine all the objectives, questions, or hypotheses?
   c. Is the treatment or intervention clearly described? Is the intervention appropriate for examining the study purpose and hypotheses? Does the study framework explain the links between the intervention (independent variable) and the proposed outcomes (dependent variables)?
   d. Was a protocol developed to promote consistent implementation of the intervention to ensure intervention fidelity (Bonar et al., 2020; Eymard & Altmiller, 2016)? Did the researcher monitor implementation of the intervention to ensure consistency? If the intervention was not consistently implemented, what might be the effect on the findings?
   e. Did the researcher identify the threats to design validity (statistical conclusion validity, internal validity, construct validity, and external validity) and minimize them as much as possible? (see Chapter 8; Gray & Grove, 2021; Kazdin, 2017; Shadish et al., 2002)
   f. If more than one group is used, do the groups appear equivalent?
   g. How were the groups formed? Were the participants randomly assigned to the intervention or control group, or were the groups naturally occurring?
   h. Were the participants in the groups matched?

7. Sample, population, and setting
   a. Is the sampling method adequate to produce a representative sample?
   b. Are any participants excluded from the study because of age, socioeconomic status, or ethnicity without a sound rationale?
   c. Did the sample include an understudied population, such as the young, elderly, or a minority group?
   d. Were the sampling criteria (inclusion and exclusion) appropriate for the type of study conducted (Gray & Grove, 2021; O'Mathúna & Fineout-Overholt, 2019)?
   e. If a power analysis was conducted, were the results of the analysis clearly described and used to determine the final sample size (Aberson, 2019)? If a power analysis was not conducted, how did the researchers determine the sample size?
   f. Was the rate of refusal to participate a problem? If so, how might this weakness have influenced the findings?
   g. Is the setting used in the study appropriate?
   h. Was sample attrition a problem? If so, how might this weakness influence the final sample and the study results and findings (Aberson, 2019; Gray & Grove, 2021)?

8. Ethical considerations
   a. Were the rights of the study participants protected?
   b. Is the study ethical?

9. Measurements
   a. Do the measurement methods selected for the study adequately measure the study variables? Should additional measurement methods have been used to improve the quality of the study outcomes (Bandalos, 2018; Gray & Grove, 2021; Waltz et al., 2017)?
   b. Do the measurement methods used in the study have adequate validity and reliability? What additional reliability or validity testing is needed to improve the quality of the measurement methods (Bandalos, 2018; Bialocerkowski et al., 2010; Waltz et al., 2017)?
   c. Respond to the following questions, which are relevant to the measurement approaches used in the study:
      (1) Scales and questionnaires
         (a) Are the instruments clearly described?
         (b) Are techniques to complete and score the instruments provided?
         (c) Are validity and reliability of the instruments described from previous research?
         (d) Did the researcher examine the reliability of instruments for the present sample?
         (e) If the instrument was developed for the study, is the instrument development process described (Bandalos, 2018; DeVellis, 2017; Waltz et al., 2017)?

  (2) Observation
    (a) Is what is to be observed clearly identified and defined?
    (b) Is interrater reliability described?
    (c) Are the techniques for recording observations described (Waltz et al., 2017)?
  (3) Structured interviews
    (a) Do the interview questions address concerns expressed in the research problem?
    (b) Are the interview questions relevant for the research purpose and objectives, questions, or hypotheses (Dillman et al., 2014; Waltz et al., 2017)?
  (4) Physiological measures
    (a) Are the physiological measures or instruments clearly described (Ryan-Wenger, 2017)? If appropriate, are the brand names, such as Space Labs or Hewlett-Packard, of the instruments identified?
    (b) Are the physiological measures appropriate for the research purpose and objectives, questions, or hypotheses?
    (c) Are the accuracy, precision, and error of the physiological instruments discussed (Ryan-Wenger, 2017)?
    (d) Are the methods for recording data from the physiological measures clearly described? Is the recording of data consistent (Gray & Grove, 2021)?

10. Data collection
  a. Is the data collection process clearly described (Gray & Grove, 2021)?
  b. Are the forms used to collect data organized to facilitate computerizing the data?
  c. Is the training of data collectors clearly described and adequate?
  d. Is the data collection process conducted in a consistent manner?
  e. Are the data collection methods ethical?
  f. Do the data collected address the research objectives, questions, or hypotheses?
  g. Did any adverse events occur during data collection; if so, were these appropriately managed?

11. Data analysis
  a. Are data analysis procedures appropriate for the type of data collected (Grove & Cipher, 2020; Kim et al., 2022; Leedy & Ormrod, 2019)?
  b. Did the researcher address any problems with missing data and how they were managed?
  c. Do the data analysis techniques address the study purpose or the research objectives, questions, or hypotheses? Are data analysis procedures clearly described?
  d. Are the results presented in an understandable way by narrative, tables, or figures, or a combination of methods (APA, 2020)?
  e. Is the sample size sufficient to detect significant differences or relationships if they are present?
  f. Was a power analysis conducted for nonsignificant results (Aberson, 2019)?
  g. Are the results interpreted appropriately?

12. Interpretation of findings
  a. Are findings discussed in relation to each objective, question, or hypothesis?
  b. Are various explanations for significant and nonsignificant findings examined?
  c. Are the findings clinically important (O'Mathúna & Fineout-Overholt, 2019)?
  d. Are the findings linked to the study framework (Smith & Liehr, 2018)?
  e. Are the findings consistent with the findings of previous studies in this area?
  f. Does the study have limitations not identified by the researcher?
  g. Did the researcher generalize the findings appropriately?
  h. Were the identified implications for practice appropriate based on the study findings and the findings from previous research (Melnyk & Fineout-Overholt, 2019)?
  i. Were quality suggestions made for future research?
  j. Do the conclusions fit the findings from this study and previous studies?

Step 3: Evaluating the Credibility and Meaning of Quantitative Study Findings

Using the following questions as a guide, summarize your evaluation of the study and document your responses.

1. Do the findings from this study build on the findings of previous studies? Review the Discussion section of the study and read some of the other relevant studies cited by the researchers to address this question.

2. When the findings are examined in light of previous studies, what is now known and not known about the phenomenon under study?

3. Could the limitations of the study have been corrected?

4. Do you believe the study findings are valid? How much confidence can be placed in the study findings (Gray & Grove, 2021)?

5. To what populations can the findings be generalized (Kazdin, 2017; Shadish et al., 2002)?

6. Are the findings ready for use in practice (Melnyk & Fineout-Overholt, 2019)?

7. What is your expert opinion of the study's quality and contribution to nursing knowledge and practice?

CRITICAL APPRAISAL GUIDELINES FOR QUALITATIVE RESEARCH

Step 1: Guidelines for Identifying the Components of the Qualitative Research Process in Studies

1. Introduction
   a. Was the article title clear?
   b. Does the title indicate the phenomenon of interest and design of the study conducted—phenomenology, grounded theory, ethnography, or exploratory-descriptive qualitative research (APA, 2020; Creswell & Poth, 2018; Gray & Grove, 2021)?
   c. Did the abstract include the purpose, sample, key results, and conclusions (APA, 2020)?

2. State the problem.
   a. Did the researchers describe the significance of the problem and/or its importance to nursing practice?
   b. Did the researchers provide the background of the problem?
   c. Was there a clear problem statement (see Chapter 5)?

3. State the purpose.
   a. Were research objectives used to guide the study?
   b. Was there an overall research question?

4. Examine the literature review.
   a. Does the review include a description of a theory and previous studies?
   b. Are the references current? (Number and percentage of sources in the last 10 years and in the last 5 years?) (see Chapter 6; Jones et al., 2020)

5. Examine the philosophical foundation or theoretical perspective of the study.
   a. Is the philosophy that supports the research design described?
   b. Was a theoretical perspective described?

6. Sampling
   a. Were inclusion and exclusion criteria identified (see Chapter 9)?
   b. How many participants were in the sample?
   c. Did the researchers identify the specific type of sampling that was used, such as purposive, network, convenience, or theoretical sampling (see Chapter 9)? If more than one type of sampling was used, did the researchers identify how many participants were recruited through each type of sampling?

7. Identify the ethical considerations.
   a. Was the study reviewed by an institutional or ethical board?
   b. What was the process for informed consent?

8. Data collection
   a. What methods were used to collect data: Interviews, focus groups, observation, or examination of documents?
   b. Did the researchers describe how data were managed and analyzed?

9. Results
   a. How were the participants described—age, marital status, or other relevant demographic variables?
   b. Were the results of the analysis presented as themes, concepts, or a diagram?

10. Discussion
    a. What were the findings of the study? Identify two findings discussed by the researchers.
    b. What study limitations did the researcher identify?
    c. Did the researcher indicate whether the findings might be applicable to other samples?
    d. What were the implications of the findings for nursing practice, if any?
    e. What suggestions for further study were identified?

11. Conclusions
    a. What conclusions did the researchers identify?

CRITICAL APPRAISAL GUIDELINES

Step 2: Determining the Strengths and Weaknesses of Qualitative Studies

1. Research problem and purpose
   a. Is the problem significant for nursing (Gallagher-Ford et al., 2020; Meadows-Oliver, 2019)?
   b. Does the purpose fit the research problem (Leedy & Ormond, 2019)?

2. Review of literature
   a. Is the literature review organized to demonstrate the progressive development of evidence from previous research (Creswell & Creswell, 2018; Leedy & Ormond., 2019)?
   b. Does the summary of the literature review identify what is known and not known about the research problem and provide direction for the formation of the purpose (Grainger, 2021)?

3. Study framework: Philosophical and theoretical foundations
   a. Was the philosophical foundation or theory appropriate for the research design (Creswell & Poth, 2018)?
   b. If a theory guided the study, was it appropriate for the phenomenon of interest and study purpose and used to guide the research questions and data analysis (Creswell, & Poth, 2018; Meadows-Oliver, 2019)?

4. Research objectives, questions, or hypotheses
   a. Were the objectives and questions expressed clearly and consistent with the study design (Gray & Grove, 2021)?
   b. Were the objectives and questions logically linked to the study results (Leedy & Ormrod, 2019; O'Sullivan & Jefferson, 2020)?

5. Design
   a. Was the design consistent with the philosophical foundation of the study (Creswell & Creswell, 2018; Creswell & Poth, 2018)?
   b. Was the design consistent with the purpose and research question (Leedy & Ormrod, 2019)?

6. Sampling and the researcher–participant relationship
   a. Were the participants' characteristics and life experiences appropriate to the qualitative approach (see Chapter 3)?
   b. Was the number of participants adequate to fulfill the purpose of the study (Creswell & Poth, 2018)?
   c. Were the length and depth of the researcher–participant relationships in the study appropriate to the study approach and study purpose (Seidman, 2019)?

7. Ethical considerations
   a. Were the rights of the study participants protected (see Chapter 4)?
   b. Was the data collection conducted in a safe and private setting (Creswell & Creswell, 2018)?

8. Data collection
   For the data collection methods used in the study, answer the following questions:
   a. Interviews
      (1) Do the interview questions address concerns expressed in the research problem?
      (2) Are the interview questions relevant for the research purpose and objectives or questions?
      (3) Were the interviews adequate in length and number to address the research purpose or answer the research question (see Chapter 3; Seidman, 2019)?
   b. Focus groups
      (1) Were the size, composition, and length of the focus group adequate to promote group interaction and to produce robust data (Creswell & Poth, 2018; Kamberelis et al., 2018)?
      (2) Were questions used during the focus group relevant to the study's research purpose and objectives or questions (Gray & Grove, 2021; Seidman, 2019)?
   c. Observation
      (1) Did the researcher provide details about how much time was spent in observation, including at what times of the day, on which days of the week, and the cumulative amount of time spent (Leedy & Ormrod, 2019)?
      (2) Did the researcher describe how notes were made about the observations, such as were notes made during the observation or after the observation (Creswell & Poth, 2018)?
      (3) Were the observations of adequate length and implemented across days and times to provide rich data related to the study purpose (Leedy & Ormrod, 2019)?
   d. Examining documents and media as data
      (1) Were the documents or media materials created specifically for the study, such as participants' textual responses to a series of open-ended questions on a questionnaire?
      (2) For materials not created for the study, were their authenticity and authorship confirmed, such as policy documents and information on websites (Decker et al., 2021)?

9. Data management, analysis, and interpretation
   a. Were data analysis and interpretation consistent with the philosophical orientation, research problem, methodology, research question, and purpose of the study (Creswell & Poth, 2018; Miles et al., 2020)?
   b. Did the researchers describe how they recorded decisions made during analysis and interpretation, usually in the form of an audit trail (Miles et al., 2020)?
   c. Did the researchers link the codes and themes used with participants' quotes?
   d. Did the researchers provide adequate description of the data analysis and interpretation processes (Miles et al., 2020)?

10. Results
    a. Were the results presented in a way that was consistent with the qualitative design and philosophy (Creswell & Poth, 2018)?
       (1) Phenomenology—rich description of live experience
       (2) Grounded theory—theoretical description of social processes
       (3) Ethnography—description of a culture, whether race/ethnic or an organization
       (4) Exploratory-descriptive qualitative research—problem-solving answer to the research question
    b. Were the results supported by participant quotes, specific observations, or analysis of the documents (Miles et al., 2020; O'Sullivan & Jefferson, 2020)?

11. Discussion
    a. Are findings discussed in relation to the objectives or questions?
    b. Are the findings linked to the study framework or philosophical foundation (Smith & Liehr, 2018)?
    c. Are the findings consistent with the findings of previous studies in this area (Creswell & Creswell, 2018)?
    d. Does the study have limitations not identified by the researcher?
    e. Were the identified implications for practice appropriate based on the study findings and the findings from previous research (Melnyk & Fineout-Overholt, 2019)?

    f.   Were quality suggestions made for future research?

    g.   Do the conclusions fit the findings from this study and previous studies?

CRITICAL APPRAISAL GUIDELINES

Step 3: Evaluating the Trustworthiness and Meaning of Qualitative Study Findings

1.   Do the study findings accurately portray the perspectives of the participants (Stahl & King, 2020)?

2.   Were standards of qualitative research applied during the study, such as the detail built into the design, carefulness of data collection, and thoroughness of analysis (Creswell & Creswell, 2018; Morse, 2018)?

3.   Do the findings from this study build on the findings of previous studies?

4.   When the findings are integrated with the findings of previous studies, what is now known and not known about the phenomenon under study?

5.   Could the limitations of the study have been corrected?

6.   Do you believe the study findings are trustworthy and credible? How much confidence can be placed in the study findings (Gray & Grove, 2021; Meadows-Oliver, 2019)?

7.   What is your overall evaluation of the study's quality and contribution to nursing knowledge and practice?

NOTES

NOTES

NOTES

NOTES

NOTES

NOTES